Advances in Anatomy, Embryology and Cell Biology
Ergebnisse der Anatomie und Entwicklungsgeschichte
Revues d'anatomie et de morphologie expérimentale
Springer-Verlag Berlin Heidelberg New York

This journal publishes reviews and critical articles covering the entire field of normal anatomy (cytology, histology, cyto- and histochemistry, electron microscopy, macroscopy, experimental morphology and embryology and comparative anatomy). Papers dealing with anthropology and clinical morphology will also be accepted with the aim of encouraging co-operation between anatomy and related disciplines.

Papers, which may be in English, French or German, are normally commissioned, but original papers and communications may be submitted and will be considered so long as they deal with a subject comprehensively and meet the requirements of the Ergebnisse.

For speed of publication and breadth of distribution, this journal appears in single issues which can be purchased separately; 6 issues constitute one volume.

It is a fundamental condition that manuscripts submitted should not have been published elsewhere, in this or any other country, and the author must undertake not to publish elsewhere at a later date.

25 copies of each paper are supplied free of charge.

Les résultats publient des sommaires et des articles critiques concernant l'ensemble du domaine de l'anatomie normale (cytologie, histologie, cyto et histochimie, microscopie électronique, macroscopie, morphologie expérimentale, embryologie et anatomie comparée. Seront publiés en outre les articles traitant de l'anthropologie et de la morphologie clinique, en vue d'encourager la collaboration entre l'anatomie et les disciplines voisines.

Seront publiés en priorité les articles expressément demandés nous tiendrons toutefois compte des articles qui nous seront envoyés dans la mesure où ils traitent d'un sujet dans son ensemble et correspondent aux standards des «Résultats». Les publications seront faites en langues anglaise, allemande et française.

Dans l'intérêt d'une publication rapide et d'une large diffusion les travaux publiés paraitront dans des cahiers individuels, diffusés séparément: 6 cahiers formen t un volume.

En principe, seuls les manuscrits qui n'ont encore été publiés ni dans le pays d'origine ni à l'étranger peuvent nous être soumis. L'auteur d'engage en outre à ne pas les publier ailleurs ultérieurement.

Les auteurs recevront 25 exemplaires gratuits de leur publication.

Die Ergebnisse dienen der Veröffentlichung zusammenfassender und kritischer Artikel aus dem Gesamtgebiet der normalen Anatomie (Cytologie, Histologie, Cyto- und Histochemie, Elektronenmikroskopie, Makroskopie, experimentelle Morphologie und Embryologie und vergleichende Anatomie). Aufgenommen werden ferner Arbeiten anthropologischen und morphologisch-klinischen Inhaltes, mit dem Ziel, die Zusammenarbeit zwischen Anatomie und Nachbardisziplinen zu fördern.

Zur Veröffentlichung gelangen in erster Linie angeforderte Manuskripte, jedoch werden auch eingesandte Arbeiten und Orginalmitteilungen berücksichtigt, sofern sie ein Gebiet umfassend abhandeln und den Anforderungen der ,,Ergebnisse" genügen. Die Veröffentlichungen erfolgen in englischer, deutscher und französischer Sprache.

Die Arbeiten erscheinen im Interesse einer raschen Veröffentlichung und einer weiten Verbreitung als einzeln berechnete Hefte; je 6 Hefte bilden einen Band.

Grundsätzlich dürfen nur Manuskripte eingesandt werden, die vorher weder im Inland noch im Ausland veröffentlicht worden sind. Der Autor verpflichtet sich, sie auch nachträglich nicht an anderen Stellen zu publizieren.

Die Mitarbeiter erhalten von ihren Arbeiten zusammen 25 Freiexemplare.

Manuscripts should be addressed to/Envoyer les manuscrits à/Manuskripte sind zu senden an:

Prof. Dr. A. BRODAL, Universitetet i Oslo, Anatomisk Instituut, Karl Johans Gate 47 (Domus Media), Oslo 1/Norwegen

Prof. W. HILD, Department of Anatomy. The University of Texas Medical Branch, Galveston, Texas 77550 (USA)

Prof. Dr. J. van LIMBORGH, Universiteit van Amsterdam, Anatomisch-Embryologisch Laboratorium, Amsterdam-O/Holland, Mauritskade 61

Prof. Dr. R. ORTMANN, Anatomisches Institut der Universität, D-5000 Köln-Lindenthal, Lindenburg

Prof. Dr. T. H. SCHIEBLER, Anatomisches Institut der Universität, Koellikerstraße 6, D-8700 Würzburg

Prof. Dr. G. TÖNDURY, Direktion der Anatomie, Gloriastraße 19, CH-8006 Zürich

Prof. Dr. E. WOLFF, Collège de France, Laboratoire d'Embryologie Expérimentale, 49 bis Avenue de la belle Gabrielle, Nogent-sur-Marne 94/France

Advances in Anatomy, Embryology and Cell Biology
Ergebnisse der Anatomie und Entwicklungsgeschichte
Revues d'anatomie et de morphologie expérimentale

47 · 5

Editors

A. Brodal, Oslo · W. Hild, Galveston · J. van Limborgh, Amsterdam ·
R. Ortmann, Köln · T. H. Schiebler, Würzburg · G. Töndury, Zürich ·
E. Wolff, Paris

Ennio Pannese

The Histogenesis of the Spinal Ganglia

With 25 Figures

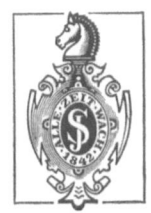

Springer-Verlag Berlin Heidelberg GmbH 1974

Prof. Dr. Ennio Pannese
Università degli Studi di Milano —2° Istituto di Anatomia Umana
Via Mangiagalli, 31
20133 Milano (Italy)

ISBN 978-3-540-06343-8   ISBN 978-3-662-10338-8 (eBook)
DOI 10.1007/978-3-662-10338-8

© by Springer-Verlag Berlin Heidelberg 1974

Originally published by Springer-Verlag Berlin Heidelberg New York in 1974.

Library of Congress Catalog Card Number 73-81288.

Printed by H. Stürtz AG, Universitätsdruckerei, D-8700 Würzburg, Germany.

To my Father, and
to the memory of my Mother

Contents

I. Introduction

The present review is based on the data of the literature, and on the personal experience gained by the author in recent years by studying the histogenesis of spinal ganglia. Probably, the reader will find more than one gap in the bibliography. The author would like to point out that in no case are such gaps due to the voluntary omission of any information, interpretations, or views. The gaps are due only to the difficulties met in trying to master such a vast literature consisting of so many contributions which have appeared over more than a century.

An endeavour has been made to report not only the morphological data, but also, whenever possible, information derived from histochemical and biochemical studies.

II. Origin of the Spinal Ganglia

Before 1868 it was generally thought (see, e.g., Remak, 1851; Bidder and Küpffer, 1857) that the spinal ganglia arise from the mesoblast of the protovertebrae (old term for somites). In 1868 His showed that the nerve cells of the spinal ganglia take their origin from the ectoderm, and more precisely from a thin band of ectoderm (Zwischenstrang, neural crest) flanking each side of the neural plate (Fig. 1 a) and interposed between it and the somatic ectoderm (Hornblatt). On this subject His (1879) wrote in a later paper "... die spinalen Ganglien ... aus einem schmalen Substanzstreifen hervorgehen, welche zwischen der Medullarplatte und dem Hornblatte gelegen ist und dessen Material ich als Zwischenstrang bezeichnet habe".

The ectodermal origin of the spinal ganglia neurons was then confermed by Balfour (1876), Marshall (1877, 1878), Onodi (1884), Beard (1889), Lenhossék (1891), although some discrepancies persisted between the views of these authors. While Beard (1889), in fact, despite the polemic spirit of his article, agreed substantially with His' view, namely that "the spinal ganglia of Vertebrates are formed as differentiations ... of the epiblast just outside the limits of the neural plate", Balfour (1876), Marshall (1877), and Onodi (1884) held that the spinal ganglia take their origin from cells coming from the neural tube proper.

The first experimental evidence that the spinal ganglia are derivatives of the neural crest was offered by Harrison (1904, 1924). In frog embryos he excised the dorsal part of the trunk, including the dorsal half of the neural tube, immediately after the closure of the neural folds, thus obtaining larvae lacking spinal ganglia. Similar results were produced in the chicken by Müller and Ingvar (1923) and in Amblystoma punctatum by DuShane (1938).

At the time of closure of the neural tube and fusion of the somatic ectoderm from both sides on the dorsal midline, the neural crest separates from the somatic ectoderm and appears as a column of cells along the dorsal aspect of the neural tube (Fig. 1 c). But the cells of the neural crest soon leave this position

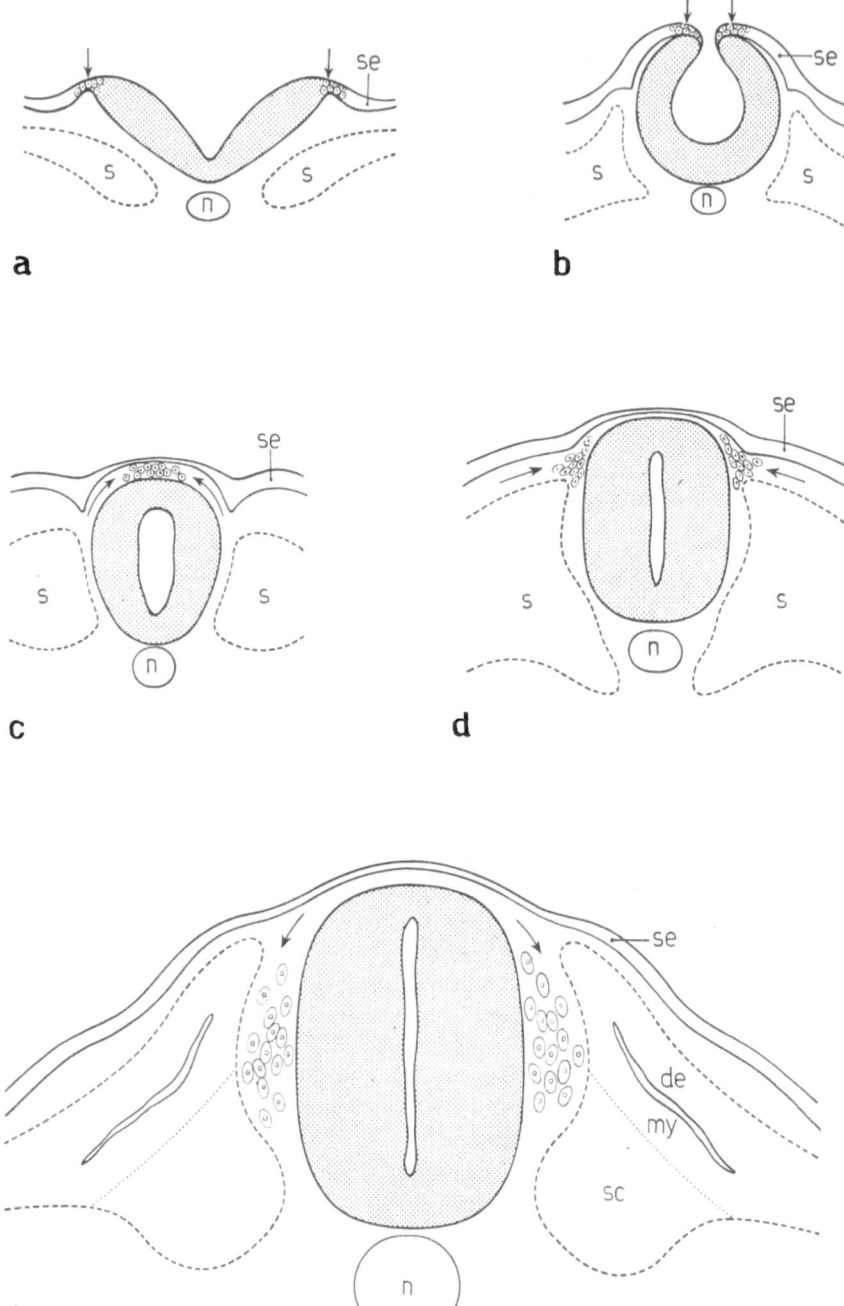

Fig. 1 a–e. Diagram showing stages in the development of spinal ganglia from the neural crest (transverse sections of five successively older, a–e, chick embryos). In Fig. a–c arrows point to the neural crest, in Fig. d and e arrows point to migrating crest cells. The neural groove and the neural tube are shown stippled. *de* dermatome, *my* myotome; *n* notochord, *s* somite, *sc* sclerotome, *se* somatic ectoderm

by migrating in a lateral and ventral direction, and they come to lie along the dorso-lateral aspect of the neural tube (Fig. 1 d). The neural crest forms and its cells begin to migrate generally in an anterior to posterior sequence along the length of the embryonic axis. Therefore, various stages of neural crest formation and migration exist at the same time in a single embryo.

In the early developmental stages the neural crest appears as a unitary structure and does not show any segmentation (Lenhossék, 1891; Harrison, 1901). Afterwards some migrating crest cells gather in small groups serially arranged along the lateral aspect of the spinal cord (Fig. 1 e). These groups represent the rudiments of the spinal ganglia. The experiments of Lehmann (1927) and Detwiler (1934) have shown that the serial arrangement of the spinal ganglia is dependent on the metamerism of the somites. In a more general sense, the influence of the surrounding tissues on the maturation of the embryonic spinal ganglia has been shown by the results of Peterson and Murray (1955).

The other cells of the neural crest are soon scattered throughout the body and thus differentiate according to various lines; therefore within a short time the neural crest disappears.

As to the origin of satellite cells, up to the end of the last century many authors regarded these cells as originating from mesenchymal elements which enter the ganglionic rudiment after its formation (His, 1890; Morpurgo and Tirelli, 1893; Kolster, 1899; Bardeen, 1903). Other authors, however, claimed that nerve and satellite cells of the spinal ganglia share a common ectodermal origin (Dohrn, 1891; Kölliker, 1905; Streeter, 1905, 1912; Kohn, 1907; Lenhossék, 1907; Levi, 1907, 1908; Held, 1909). Streeter (1905) and Lenhossék (1907) held that all the cells of the rudiment of the spinal ganglion show at first the same morphological characteristics, then they differentiate along two lines, some becoming ganglionic neurons, others satellite cells. The experimental researches of Harrison (1904), Detwiler (1937), and Jones (1939) speak in favour of the neural crest as the source of the satellite cells of the spinal ganglia, while Kuntz' (1922) and Raven's (1937) findings disagree with those of the above authors. It is widespread belief now, that the satellite cells of spinal ganglia arise from the neural crest while those of the sympathetic ganglia would arise in part from the neural crest and in part from the neural tube (Brizzee, 1949).

The rudiments of spinal ganglia increase rapidly in volume. This increase is due at the beginning to the recruitment of additional migrating cells moving away from the neural crest and to the proliferation of the cells which have reached their final position in the ganglia (see chapter III). Later, the increase in volume of the spinal ganglia depends to a large extent on the gradual and considerable growth of the cell body of the individual elements which differentiate into neuroblasts and then develop into mature nerve cells (see chapter IV). Finally, the increase in number of the satellite cells and the development of interstitial spaces and blood vessels (see chapter VI) contribute to the further increase in volume of the spinal ganglia.

III. Undifferentiated Cells

In the spinal ganglia of the chick embryo the undifferentiated cells are numerous in early developmental stages, when they often appear arranged in small groups.

Later, their relative number differs in the lateroventral and the mediodorsal region of the ganglion respectively. In the lateroventral part of the ganglion (where the neurons differentiate early) the undifferentiated cells soon become relatively scarce, and they are found scattered singly among the neuroblasts. Instead, in the mediodorsal part of the ganglion the undifferentiated cells remain numerous throughout the first half of the incubation period, being particularly located close to the ganglion surface.

At the light microscope level the undifferentiated cells appear rounded or polyhedral with short expansions (Fig. 3a). The nucleus is ovoid or spherical, rich in chromatin.

At the electron microscope level (Fig. 2a) the cytoplasmic rim appears to contain clusters of free[1] ribosomes in each section, and small, rough-surfaced cisternae in single sections only. The Golgi complex appears poorly developed; seldom, in fact, a section of the Golgi complex built of a few, small cisternae and some associated vesicles can be seen. Mitochondria are scarce; many sections of undifferentiated cells do not contain, in fact, mitochondrial profiles; only in some sections one to three mitochondrial profiles can be seen. Individual microtubules are scattered in the cytoplasmic rim, while filaments are not evident. Rarely a cilium is found which projects into a channel formed by a deep invagination of the plasma membrane. The chromatin appears rather condensed in the undifferentiated cell nucleus. The nucleolus often shows a more compact texture in respect to that of other ganglionic cells.

Adhering and/or gap junctions sometimes link the undifferentiated to adjacent cells.

Undifferentiated cells can often be observed in mitosis. The dividing undifferentiated cells retain the junctions with adjacent cells, as was observed also in the neural tube by Hinds and Ruffett (1971).

The mitotic process of undifferentiated cells will not be described here in detail, but only some structural changes occurring during mitosis will be dealt with.

During prophase, undifferentiated cells appear spherical or oval in shape and are usually devoid of expansions. While in the interphase undifferentiated cells show most of the ribosomes arranged in clusters, from prometaphase to anaphase most ribosomes occur singly or in irregular aggregates. The disaggregation or ribosomal clusters during mitosis has been described (in HeLa cells) by Scharff and Robbins (1966), who showed also that this disaggregation was accompanied

Fig. 2a and b. Undifferentiated cells. Fig. a (spinal ganglion of a chick embryo: 22000 ×) shows an undifferentiated cell whose cytoplasmic rim contains clusters of free ribosomes, some microtubules (arrows), and two small profiles of the endoplasmic reticulum. Crossed arrow points to a pinocytotic vesicle. Fig. b (spinal ganglion of a chick embryo, Karnovsky's method for AChE activity: 17500 ×; preparation by E. Pannese, L. Luciano, S. Iurato, and E. Reale) shows an undifferentiated cell whose contour is outlined in ink. Granules of the reaction product appear localized within the perinuclear cisterna of the undifferentiated cell and also within the endoplasmic reticulum cisternae (arrowed) of an adjacent neuroblast. Note that the endoplasmic reticulum cisternae in the undifferentiated cell (crossed arrows) do not contain reaction product

1 The term "free" ribosomes is referred to ribosomes (either isolated or grouped in clusters) not attached to membranes.

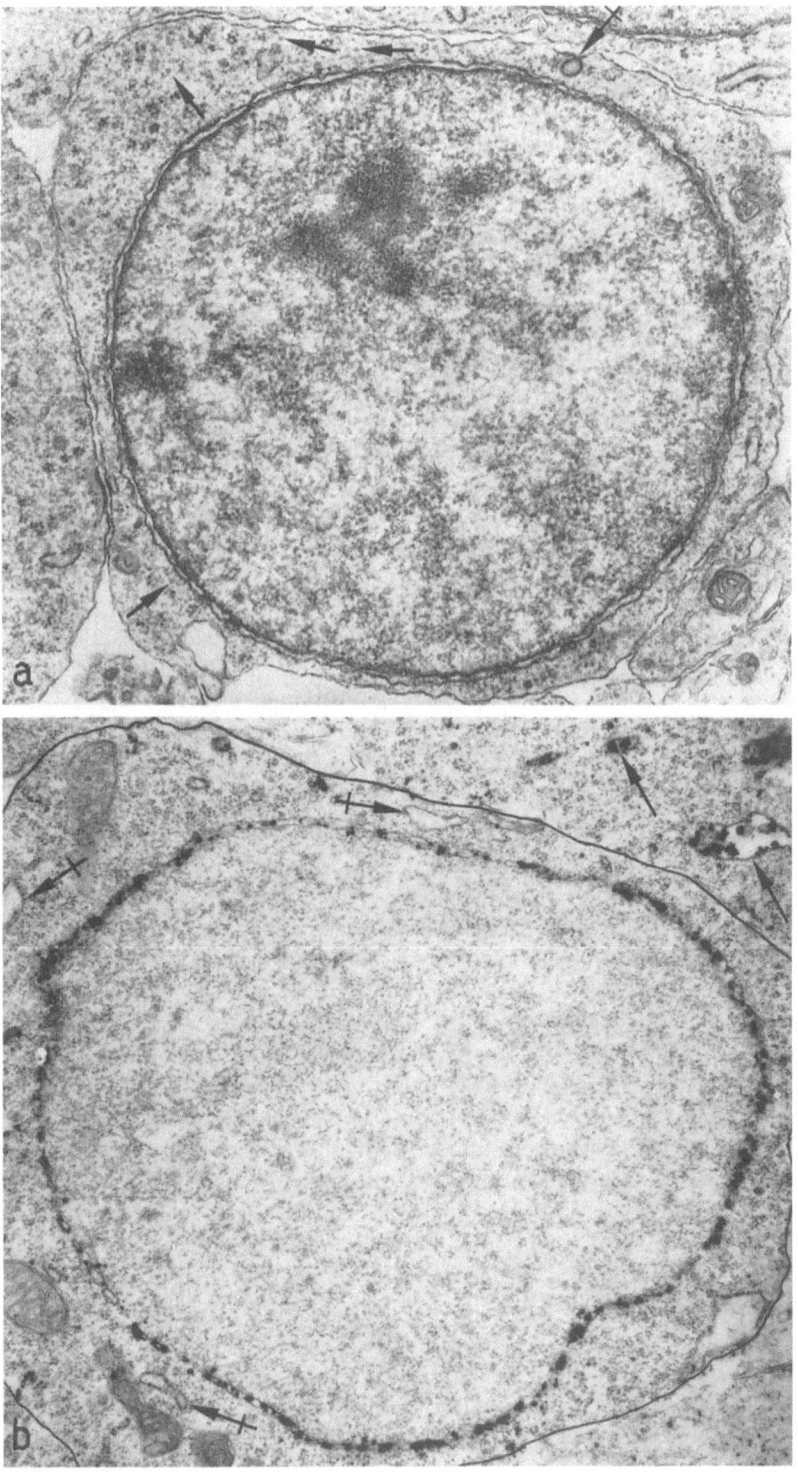

Fig. 2a and b

by a sudden decrease in protein synthesis. Long cisternae of the endoplasmic reticulum are common during metaphase in the peripheral region of the cell. They occur only rarely in apposed parallel pairs and probably represent remnants of the nuclear envelope. A small Golgi complex is sometimes evident in prophase, prometaphase, and anaphase cells. A cilium has sometimes been observed in early prophase cells, not during later phases.

IV. Development of the Nerve Cell

A. Light Microscopy

1. Cell Shape and Processes

At the beginning of the transformation to neuroblast, the short expansions of the undifferentiated cell disappear, and the cytoplasm increases in size; this transitional element may sometimes be found in mitosis. Later the cell elongates becoming spindle-shaped (Fig. 3b), and two processes grow out from the two opposite poles of the perikaryon (bipolar neuroblast, or primitive neuroblast). The bipolar form of the primitive neuroblast in spinal ganglia was first described by His (1886) and later confirmed by Cajal (1890a), Retzius (1891), and Lenhossék (1892). Of the two processes of the primitive neuroblast, the one directed toward the periphery is thicker than the one directed toward the spinal cord. The former grows in length rapidly. In the lateroventral region of the spinal ganglia of the chick embryo the primitive neuroblasts are already evident at the 3rd incubation day; they are quite numerous from the 4th to the 6th incubation day; afterwards their number decreases gradually.

As development proceeds the shape of the neuroblast changes markedly. The perikaryal cytoplasm increases in volume and becomes thicker on one side of the nucleus (Fig. 3c, d); the cell, therefore, becomes bell-shaped and at the same time the two processes gradually approach each other (intermediate neuroblast). The intermediate neuroblast was accurately described by His (1886, 1887). In the latero-ventral region of the spinal ganglia of the chick embryo these cells are sometimes detectable already during the 4th incubation day; usually they are numerous at the 5th day.

Afterwards, the cytoplasmic portion remaining between the sites of emergence of the processes elongates gradually into a thick trunk from which the processes bifurcate. Thus the cell becomes globular- or pear-shaped (Fig. 3e) with a single process (pseudo-unipolar nerve cell). In the spinal ganglia of the chick embryo the pseudo-unipolar nerve cells appear at the beginning of the second half of the incubation period. The transformation of the spinal ganglia neuroblasts from bipolar to pseudo-unipolar was first mentioned by His (1886), clearly illustrated by Cajal (1891) in a figure and later described in more detail (see Cajal, 1904).

The growing processes of the spinal ganglia neuroblasts end with growth cones. The growth cones were first described by Cajal (1890 b; see also 1909) as bulbous enlargements sending out thin membranous extensions. Afterwards Harrison (1907, 1910) and Speidel (1933) observed the growth cones in living neuroblasts, and Levi (1917), Hughes (1953), Nakai and Kawasaki (1959), Pomerat et al. (1967), and Yamada et al. (1971) described their dynamic activity in tissue cultures.

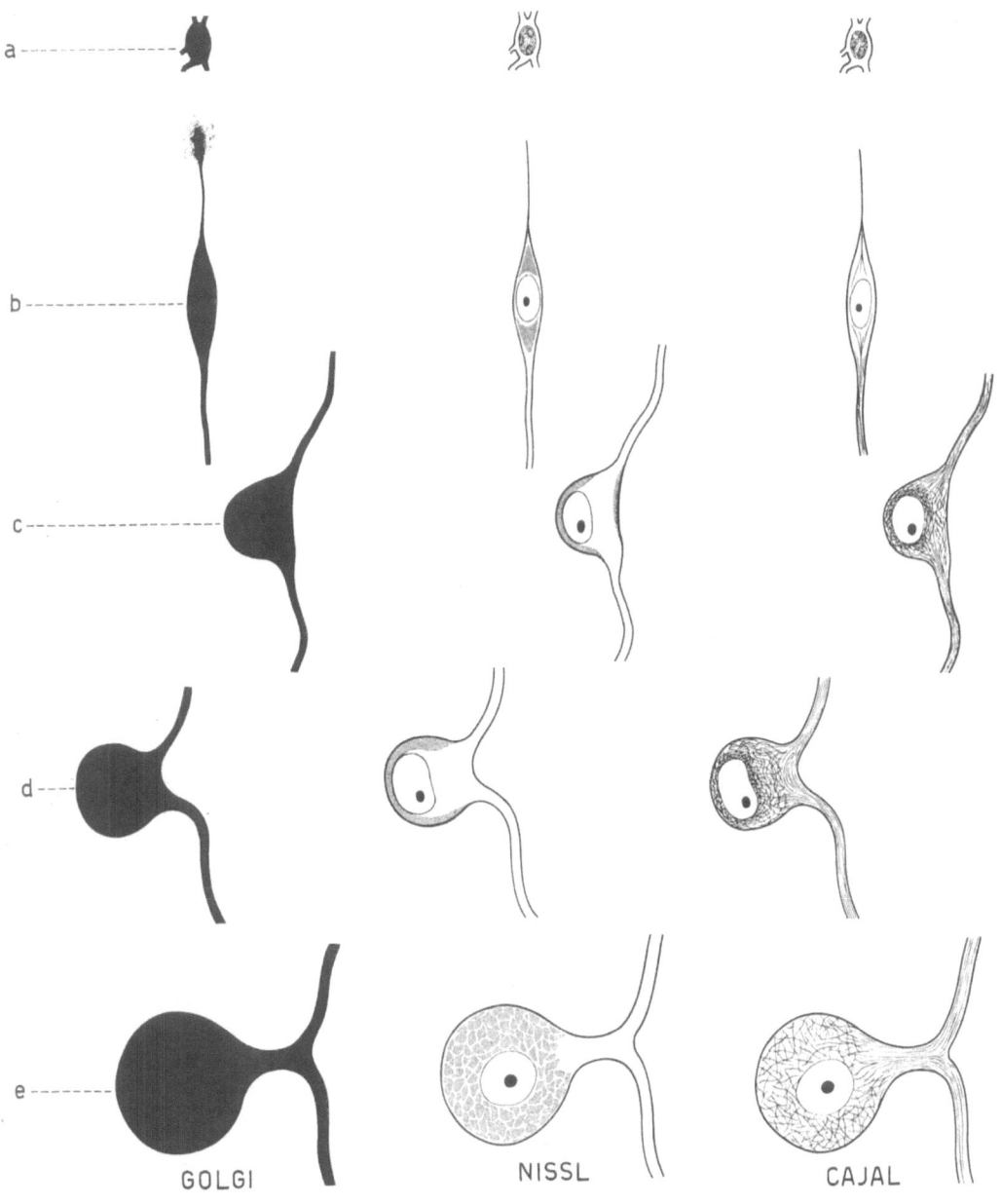

Fig. 3a–e. Diagram showing some major events occurring at the light microscope level during the differentiation and maturation of a spinal ganglion nerve cell. The Golgi's method makes evident the changes in cell shape, the Nissl's method the changes in Nissl substance, and, finally, the Cajal's silver method the changes in the neurofibrils. a, undifferentiated cell; b, primitive neuroblast; c and d, intermediate neuroblasts; e, pseudo-unipolar nerve cell

2. Nucleus

The primitive neuroblast has an ovoid nucleus, the main axis of which coincides with that of the cell (Fig. 3 b); this nucleus shows one or more large nucleoli, and the karyoplasm appears more clear than that of the undifferentiated cell nucleus. The transformation of the undifferentiated cell into a neuroblast is not characterized, therefore, only by changes in cell shape and cytoplasmic structure, but also by structural modifications of the nucleus.

The nucleus of the intermediate neuroblast (Fig. 3c, d) is often oval-shaped, eccentric, and flattened or wrinkled on the surface facing the central zone of the perikaryon (Hatai, 1904). According to Hydén (1943), nuclear eccentricity and wrinkling of the nuclear surface would be indicative of a marked synthetic activity. The pseudo-unipolar nerve cell, instead, has a central, spherical or oval nucleus (Fig. 3 e).

In the nerve cells of the sensory ganglia of the guinea pig the nucleolus develops as a light area at the edge or center of a chromocenter. Then this light area increases in size while the Feulgen-positive material assumes a peripheral position and breaks up into fine particles (LaVelle, 1956).

A change in position of the sex chromatin was observed during development of the spinal ganglion neurons in the cat. The sex chromatin appears predominantly contiguous to the nuclear envelope in early developmental stages and adjacent to the nucleolus in later developmental stages (Graham, 1954).

The nucleus/cytoplasmic ratio is very high in the undifferentiated cell, which has a very scarce cytoplasm. This ratio decreases with cell differentiation and continues to diminish gradually during the transition from the primitive neuroblast to the intermediate neuroblast, then to the pseudo-unipolar nerve cell. In fact, the cytoplasm increases in volume much more than the nucleus during these developmental stages.

3. Perikaryon

a) Nissl Substance. In the spinal ganglia of the chick embryos, Nissl substance first appears in the primitive neuroblast (Fig. 3 b) as a strongly basophilic material filling both cones of cytoplasm (Collin, 1906).

In the intermediate neuroblast (Fig. 3c, d) Nissl substance is accumulated in the peripheral region of the perikaryon (Timofeew, 1898; van Biervliet, 1900; Collin, 1906). This region shows a dense absorption in the ultraviolet at 2537 Å (Hughes, 1955). The central zone of the perikaryon instead does not stain with basic dyes. The centriole is found in this central zone (Collin, 1906).

Afterwards, the peripheral ring of Nissl substance breaks up into discrete bodies, which invade also the central zone of the perikaryon (Timofeew, 1898; van Biervliet, 1900; Collin, 1906). In this way, the Nissl substance attains its final arrangement in the pseudo-unipolar nerve cell, appearing as basophilic areas scattered at random in the perikaryon and separated by light channels (Fig. 3 e).

b) Golgi Apparatus. This organelle was first described in the neuroblasts of the ox spinal ganglia by Golgi himself (1899) then by Marcora (1911) in the chick and duck embryos. The developmental changes of the Golgi apparatus in the nerve cells of the spinal ganglia were described by Rau and Ludford (1925) and Kwan (1936). Initially, the Golgi apparatus appears as a compact cluster of rodlets situated on one side of the nucleus; successively the rodlets become scattered, branch and anastomose thus forming a perinuclear network. According to Marcora (1911) the Golgi apparatus appears earlier than the Nissl substance in the neuroblasts of the spinal ganglia of the chick and duck embryos.

   c) Neurofibrils. Neurofibrillar development during neuroblastic differentiation was studied at a later date than the Nissl substance, because neurofibrils could only be clearly visualized after improvement of impregnation methods, in particular Cajal's silver staining. Considerable difficulties were met in fact when applying Cajal's method to embryos in early stages of development.

   Besta (1904a, b) was the first to stain successfully with Cajal's method embryos at early stages of development. He noticed neurofibrils in the primitive neuroblasts of the spinal ganglia of the chick embryos already at the 3rd incubation day. At this time, in the perikaryon of these neuroblasts two neurofibrils which arrive near the nucleus from the sites of emergence of the processes can be seen (Besta, 1904a). Afterwards each of these neurofibrils branches out into 3 or 4 thinner fibrils (Fig. 3b) which encompass the nucleus (Besta, 1904b).

   According to Held (1905, 1906), the neurofibrillar differentiation begins in a special region of the neuroblast (fibrillogene Zone). Besta (1904a, b) maintains that the neurofibrils of the neuroblast are individual units which interlace, while according to Held (1905, 1906) and Marcora (1911) the neurofibrils anastomose thus forming a true network from the beginning. From the region where it first appears the neurofibrillar network spreads around the nucleus and in the neuroblastic processes.

   Changes of the neurofibrils taking place during the transformation of the primitive into the intermediate neuroblast were studied by Cajal (1904). In the primitive neuroblast at an advanced developmental stage, two neurofibrillar networks, one perinuclear and the other peripheral in position, are evident. The former is in continuity with two bundles of fibrils extending in the processes. As the two processes approach each other, also the corresponding bundles of fibrils coming from the perinuclear network draw nearer. An arched fibrillar bundle, which becomes evident afterwards, links the two bundles of fibrils lying in the processes (Fig. 3d). According to Tello (1904), the perinuclear network appears more densely packed than the peripheral one (Fig. 3c, d).

   As regards the time of appearance, Besta (1904b) and Collin (1906) maintain that the neurofibrils appear earlier than the Nissl substance in the neuroblasts of the spinal ganglia of the chick embryo (as well as in the neuroblasts of the ventral horn of the spinal cord).

4. Cell Size Changes

   In the chicken the growth rate of the nerve cells of the spinal ganglia is very high during the embryonic period, then it decreases at first rapidly and then more slowly (Olivo et al., 1932). In the rat the increase in volume of these cells is very rapid during embryonic life and the first days after birth, but is much slower between the 10th and the 30th day after birth (Sobkowicz et al., 1973). In man the nerve cells of the spinal ganglia already show an evident increase in volume during the second month of embryonic life; their growth rate is very high during the foetal period, but diminishes sharply at birth and then slowly until adult life is reached (Pilati, 1938).

The increase in volume of the nerve cells of the spinal ganglia lasts very long: in the chicken it still continues 6 months after hatching (Olivo *et al.*, 1932), and in the rat it continues up to late adult life (Donaldson and Nagasaka, 1918).

The growth of the various groups of the ganglionic nerve cells was evaluated in the chicken by Olivo *et al.* (1932). From the 6th incubation day until the 15th day after hatching the larger the cells the higher their growth rate, from the 15th day onwards after hatching the growth rate is practically the same for all ganglionic nerve cells.

B. Electron Microscopy

1. Perikaryon

a) Endoplasmic Reticulum and Ribosomes. The transitional elements between the undifferentiated cell and the primitive neuroblast (Fig. 4) have a larger peri-karyon than the undifferentiated cells almost completely filled by free ribosomal clusters (polysomes). In comparison with the undifferentiated cells, these transitional elements contain therefore a larger complement of free ribosomes.

Also the primitive neuroblasts (Figs. 6a, b, 7a, b) have a very large number of free ribosomes; they possess, as well, a prominent rough-surfaced endoplasmic reticulum (Pannese, 1968a). The development of an elaborated endoplasmic reticulum with attached polysomes is, therefore, one of the main changes which take place during the neuroblastic differentiation in the spinal ganglia. The same finding was observed by Fujita and Fujita (1963) during the differentiation of the matrix cells in the central nervous system.

In the sections of primitive neuroblasts at an early developmental stage the endoplasmic reticulum profiles are few, but very long. In these neuroblasts, the membranes of the endoplasmic reticulum may be continuous with the outer nuclear membrane (Fig. 7a, b). Sometimes in a single section and usually in the serial sections, the rough-surfaced endoplasmic reticulum appears as a system of long interconnected channels (Fig. 7a, b). The continuity of this system with the nuclear envelope is apparent in some sections only. In the sections of primitive neuroblasts at a more advanced developmental stage the endoplasmic reticulum profiles are more numerous and shorter than in the preceding stage.

Flattened, membrane-limited cisternae (subsurface cisternae, Rosenbluth, 1962) closely applied to the plasma membrane (Figs. 6a, 15d, 22a, 23) are numerous in the spinal ganglia neuroblasts (Tennyson, 1965; Pannese, 1968a; Weis, 1968). These structures have been found in all cells of the neuroblastic line. These cisternae underlie perikarya, neuroblastic processes (Fig. 6a), and satellite cells (Figs. 6a, 22a). Sometimes confronting subsurface cisternae (Figs. 15d, 23) can be seen in two adjacent cells (i.e., in two neuroblasts, or in a neuroblast and in a satellite cell). As a rule, ribosomes are not attached to the external, but to the inner aspect of the subsurface cisterna. Occasionally, subsurface cisternae appear continuous with cisternae of the rough-surfaced endoplasmic reticulum, which lie more deeply in the cell (Fig. 15d). Subsurface cisternae lacking ribosomes have also been observed, chiefly in the cell processes (Fig. 6d).

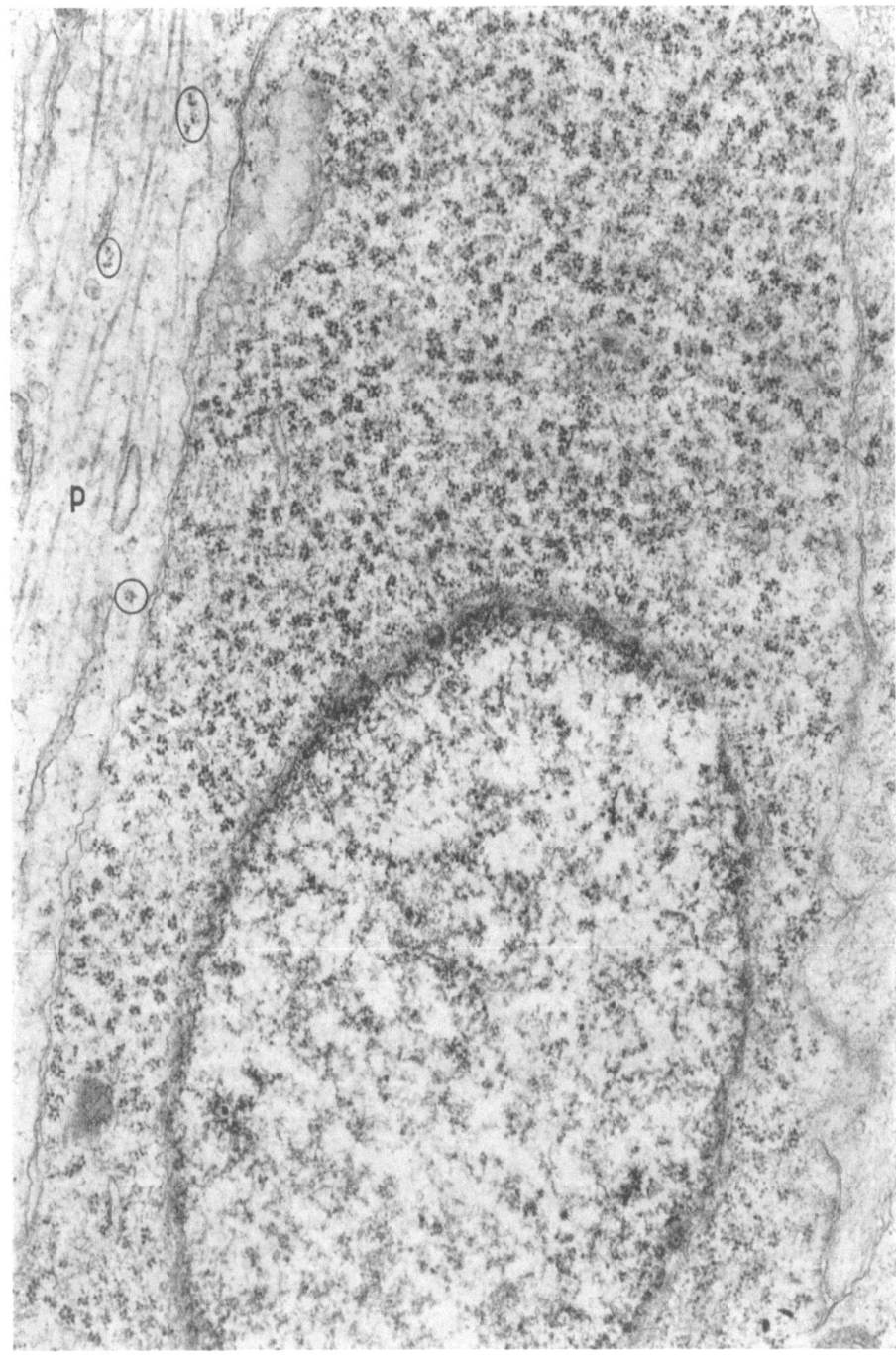

Fig. 4. Transitional element between undifferentiated cell and primitive neuroblast (spinal ganglion of a chick embryo: 30000 ×). The cytoplasm is almost completely filled by free ribosomal clusters. *p* neuroblastic process containing microtubules, rare filaments, free ribosomes (encircled), and profiles of the smooth-surfaced endoplasmic reticulum

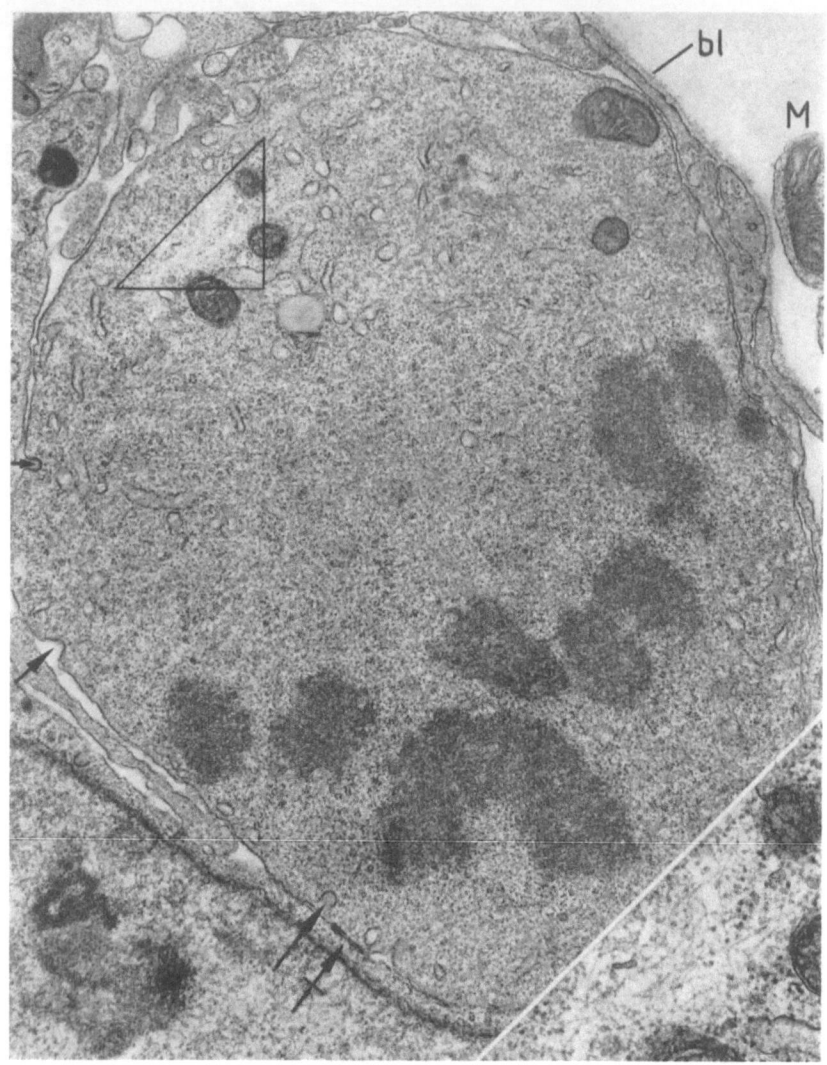

Fig. 5. Mitosis of a transitional element between undifferentiated cell and primitive neuroblast (spinal ganglion of a chick embryo: 16800 × ; inset: 40000 ×). The outlined area is enlarged in the inset to show some filaments. Arrows point to pinocytotic vesicles; crossed arrow points to a junction linking the mitotic cell to an adjacent resting cell. *bl* basal lamina which covers the contour of the ganglionic rudiment, *M* mesenchyme

Fig. 6a–e. Primitive neuroblasts (spinal ganglia of chick embryos). Fig. a (12000 ×) shows a section through the major axis of the cell body of a primitive neuroblast. A bundle of neurofilaments (encircled) can be seen in one of the perikaryal cones. Double arrow points to a subsurface cisterna underlying a satellite cell (*sc*), crossed arrow points to a subsurface cisterna underlying a neuroblastic process (*p*). The perikaryal surface of this neuroblast is partially invested by satellite cells (*sc*). Note that the satellite cell sheet intervening between two adjacent neuroblasts in the lower right consists of three adjoining cytoplasmic expansions. Arrow points to a pinocytotic vesicle in a neuroblast. (∗) indicates a degenerating cell. Fig. b (28000 ×) shows a sector of the nucleus (*N*) and an adjacent area of one of the perikaryal cones of a primitive neuroblast. Many free ribosomal clusters, profiles of the rough-surfaced endoplasmic reticulum, and a bundle of closely packed neurofilaments are evident in this cytoplasmic area. Fig. c (16000 ×) shows a sector of the nucleus (*N*) and an adjacent area of one of the perikaryal cones of a primitive neuroblast. A centriole (*c*), surrounded by Golgi complexes (*G*), is evident in this cytoplasmic area. Arrow points to a rough-surfaced profile in close proximity to the smooth-surfaced cisternae of a Golgi complex. Fig. d (24000 ×) shows a segment of the central process of a primitive neuroblast. Neurofilaments, microtubules, free

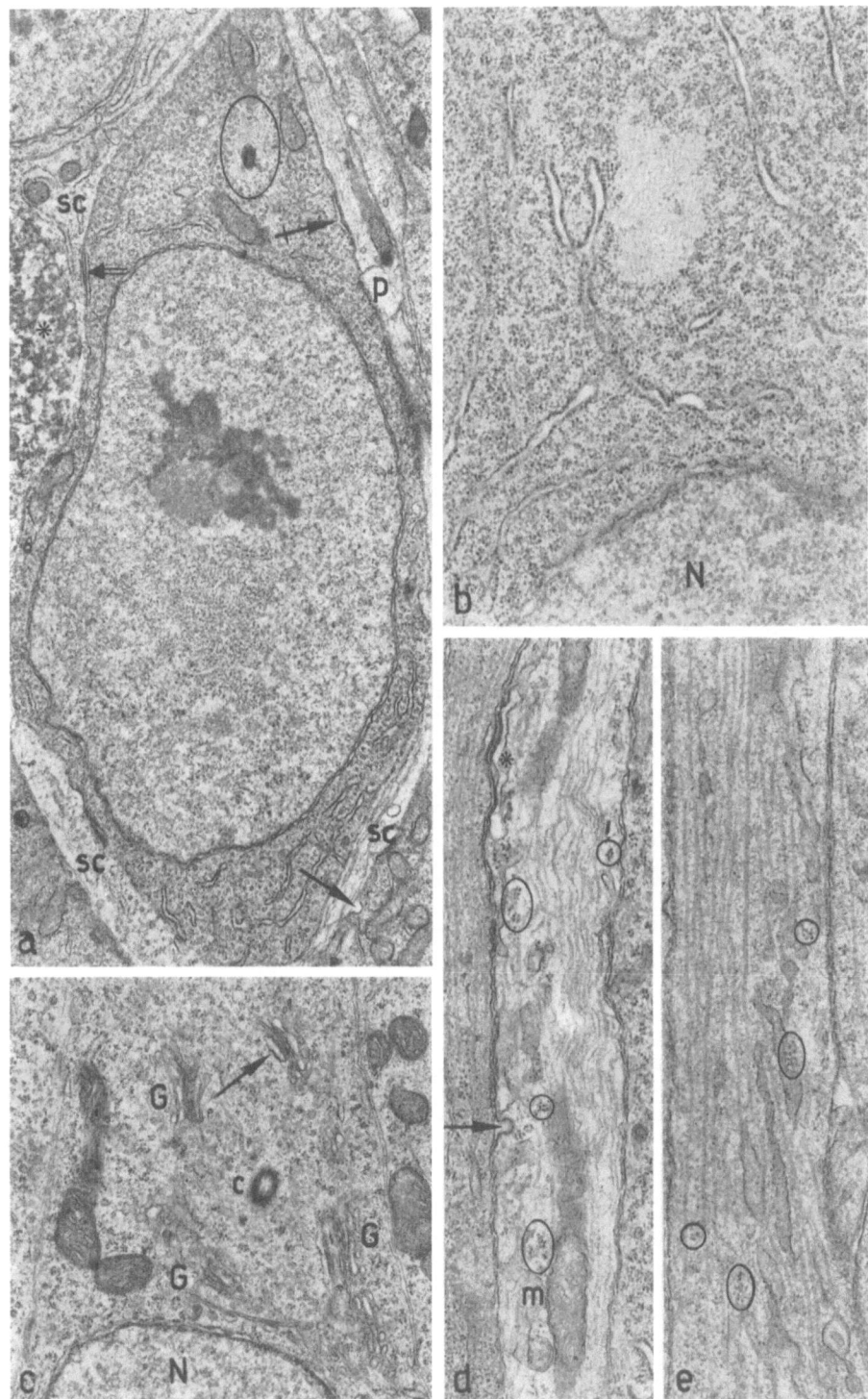

Fig. 6a–e

ribosomes (encircled), and mitochondria (m) are evident in this process. Arrow points to a pinocytotic vesicle; * indicates a subsurface cisterna lacking ribosomes. Fig. e (24000 ×) shows a segment of the peripheral process of a primitive neuroblast. Many microtubules, some neurofilaments, free ribosomes (encircled), and smooth-surfaced profiles of the endo-plasmic reticulum are evident in this process

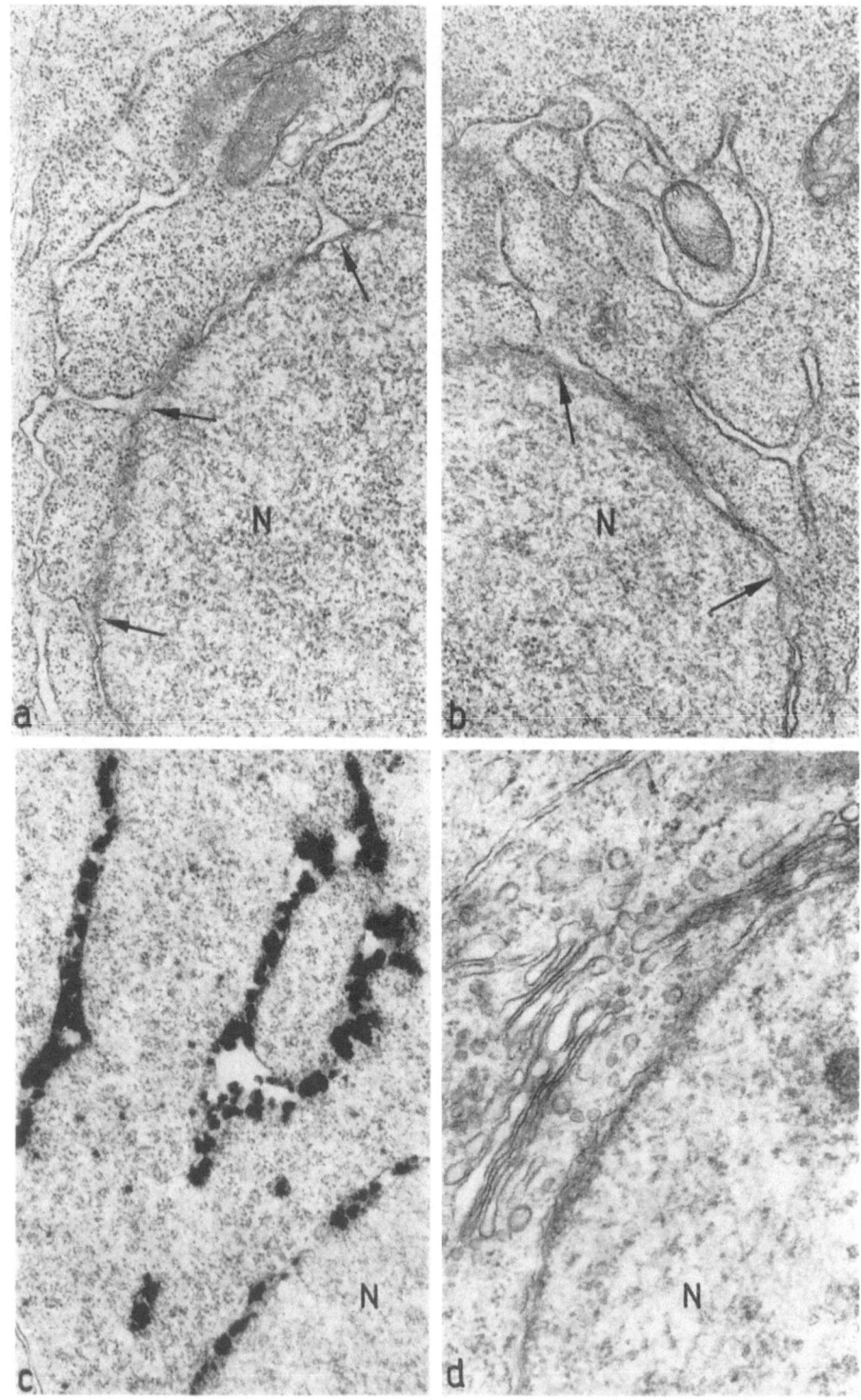

Fig. 7 a–d

In comparison with the primitive neuroblasts, the intermediate neuroblasts (Fig. 9) have a more highly developed and organized rough-surfaced endoplasmic reticulum. Most cisternae of the rough-surfaced endoplasmic reticulum and most ribosomes are confined to the peripheral region (Fig. 9) of the perikaryon (Tennyson, 1965; Pannese, 1968a), which appears strongly basophilic under the light microscope. The cisternae may be arranged in parallel arrays, more often they are distributed at random. A continuity between the rough-surfaced endoplasmic reticulum and the nuclear envelope is less frequently observed in the intermediate than in the primitive neuroblasts. It may be recalled here that the rough-surfaced endoplasmic reticulum is confined at the periphery of the perikaryon also in the pyramidal cells of Ammon's horn of the adult rabbit (Niklowitz and Bak, 1965) and in the ganglion cells of the ventral nerve cord of *Lumbricus terrestris* (Coggeshall, 1965).

In the pseudo-unipolar nerve cells (Fig. 21) the rough-surfaced endoplasmic reticulum appears localized in the Nissl bodies. Each Nissl body (Fig. 10a) appears to consist: (a) of a stack of branching cisternae, usually lacking any preferential orientation, with membranes studded with clusters of ribosomes, and (b) of free ribosomal clusters lying in the cytoplasmic matrix between the cisternae (Palay and Palade, 1955). Lighter cytoplasmic channels, containing neurofilaments, microtubules, mitochondria, and other structures intervene between the Nissl bodies. A continuity between the rough-surfaced endoplasmic reticulum and the nuclear envelope has not been detected in these cells.

Going from the primitive neuroblast to the intermediate neuroblast then to the pseudo-unipolar nerve cell, the fraction of ribosomes attached to the endoplasmic reticulum membranes steadily increases in parallel to the increase in the endoplasmic reticulum. However (see above) many free ribosomes are still present in the mature nerve cells in the cytoplasmic matrix between the cisternae of the Nissl bodies.

In all developmental stages of the nerve cell in the chick spinal ganglia both free and membrane-attached ribosomes appear steadily arranged in polysomal clusters (Pannese, 1968a). In tangentially cut cisternae, the membrane-attached ribosomes are more frequently arranged in spirals and loops than in curved or double rows; the maximum number of ribosomes in the membrane-attached polysomes is at least 13 (Pannese, 1968a). Shorter polysomes may

Fig. 7a–d. Endoplasmic reticulum and Golgi complex in primitive neuroblasts at an early developmental stage. Each of the Fig. a–d shows a sector of the nucleus (*N*) and an adjacent area of the perikaryon of a primitive neuroblast. In Fig. a and b (spinal ganglion of a chick embryo: 24000 ×) the rough-surfaced endoplasmic reticulum appears as a system of interconnected channels in continuity with the nuclear envelope (at arrows). In Fig. c (spinal ganglion of a chick embryo, Karnovsky's method for AChE activity: 24000 ×; preparation by E. Pannese, L. Luciano, S. Iurato, and E. Reale) granules of the reaction product appear localized within the perinuclear cisterna and within the rough-surfaced cisternae of the endoplasmic reticulum. Fig. d (spinal ganglion of a chick embryo: 40000 ×) shows a Golgi complex in proximity to the nuclear envelope, with its cisternae arranged parallel to it. Note that the portion of the outer nuclear membrane adjacent to the Golgi complex appears devoid of ribosomes and it exhibits small blebs. Small vesicles appear located between the nuclear envelope and the cisternae of the Golgi complex

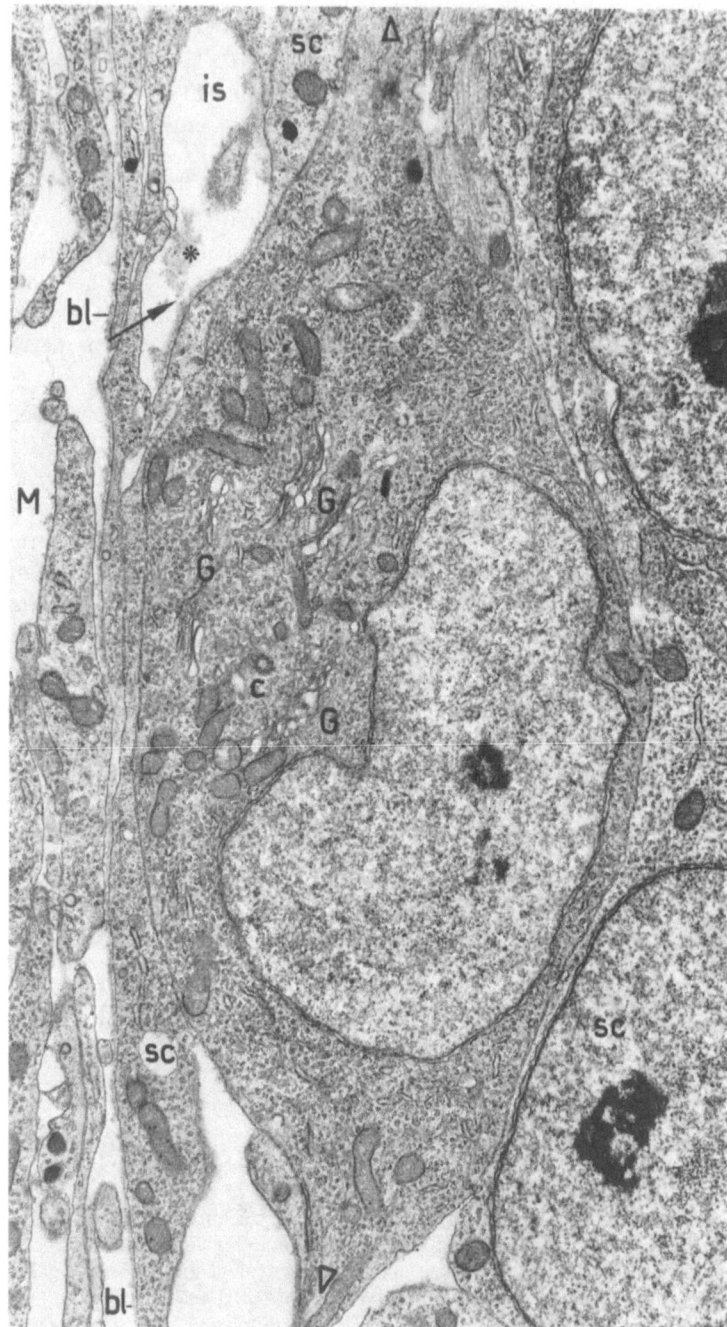

Fig. 8. Transitional cell between the primitive and intermediate neuroblast (spinal ganglion of a chick embryo: 14 000 ×). The centriole (*c*) and the Golgi complexes (*G*) lie alongside the wrinkled nuclear surface. Note that nearly all the surface of this neuroblast is invested by satellite cells (*sc*). The satellite cells (*sc*) intervene everywhere between the neuroblast and the

either represent actually shorter polysomal chains, or they may be segments of larger polysomes divided by the plane of the section. It may be recalled that the largest free polysomes obtained by Ekholm and Hydén (1965) from microdissected fresh nerve cells of the rabbit contained 12–15 ribosomes, the majority being composed of 4–5 ribosomes.

Tubules devoid of ribosomes are seldom found in the perikaryon; they are more frequently seen in the processes of the primitive neuroblasts (Figs. 4, 6e). Tubules and cisternae devoid of ribosomes are usually observed in the perikaryon of the intermediate neuroblast. Therefore, the smooth-surfaced endoplasmic reticulum appears in the perikaryon when the rough-surfaced endoplasmic reticulum is well developed. The smooth-surfaced endoplasmic reticulum appears increased in volume in the perikaryon of the pseudo-unipolar nerve cells: it consists of isolated units situated between the neurofilaments, or in continuity with the rough-surfaced cisternae in the Nissl bodies (Fig. 10a).

b) Golgi Complex. In the transitional elements between the undifferentiated cell and the primitive neuroblast, the Golgi complex is poorly developed. Very seldom, in fact, a section of the Golgi complex built of a few, small cisternae and some associated vesicles can be seen in the sections of these cells. In the primitive neuroblasts (Figs. 6c, 7d) the Golgi complex is more developed than in the above mentioned cells: in fact, a section of the Golgi complex is evident in about 1 every 3 sections of primitive neuroblasts. In these cells the Golgi complex lies in the cones of cytoplasm (Fig. 6c). Therefore, an enlargement of the Golgi complex takes place during the neuroblastic differentiation in the chick embryo spinal ganglia.

In the primitive neuroblast the Golgi complex lies sometimes in close proximity to the nuclear envelope, with its cisternae arranged parallel to it (Fig. 7d). In these cases the portion of the outer nuclear membrane adjacent to the Golgi complex appears devoid of ribosomes and it exhibits small blebs. Instead, in the intermediate neuroblast and in the pseudo-unipolar nerve cell this kind of relationship between the nuclear envelope and Golgi complex has not been observed.

In the primitive neuroblasts, rough-surfaced profiles (Fig. 6c) may be found in proximity to the smooth-surfaced cisternae of the Golgi complex (Tennyson, 1965; Pannese, 1968a). Similar findings have been pointed out by Fauré-Fremiet *et al.* (1962), and by Vivier and Schrevel (1966) in Protozoa. It has also been seen in the serial sections that the rough-surfaced cisternae close to a Golgi complex belong to an extensive and branched endoplasmic reticulum (Pannese, 1968a).

In the transitional elements between the primitive and the intermediate neuroblasts, the Golgi complex usually lies alongside the flattened or wrinkled nuclear surface (Fig. 8). In comparison with the primitive neuroblast, the intermediate

basal lamina *(bl)* which covers the contour of the ganglionic rudiment. An interstitial space *(is)*, bordered by satellite cells, is evident (top left). This space contains a patch of moderately dense material (✱), which at arrow appears in contact with a primordium of the basal lamina. *M* mesenchyme. △ indicates cell processes

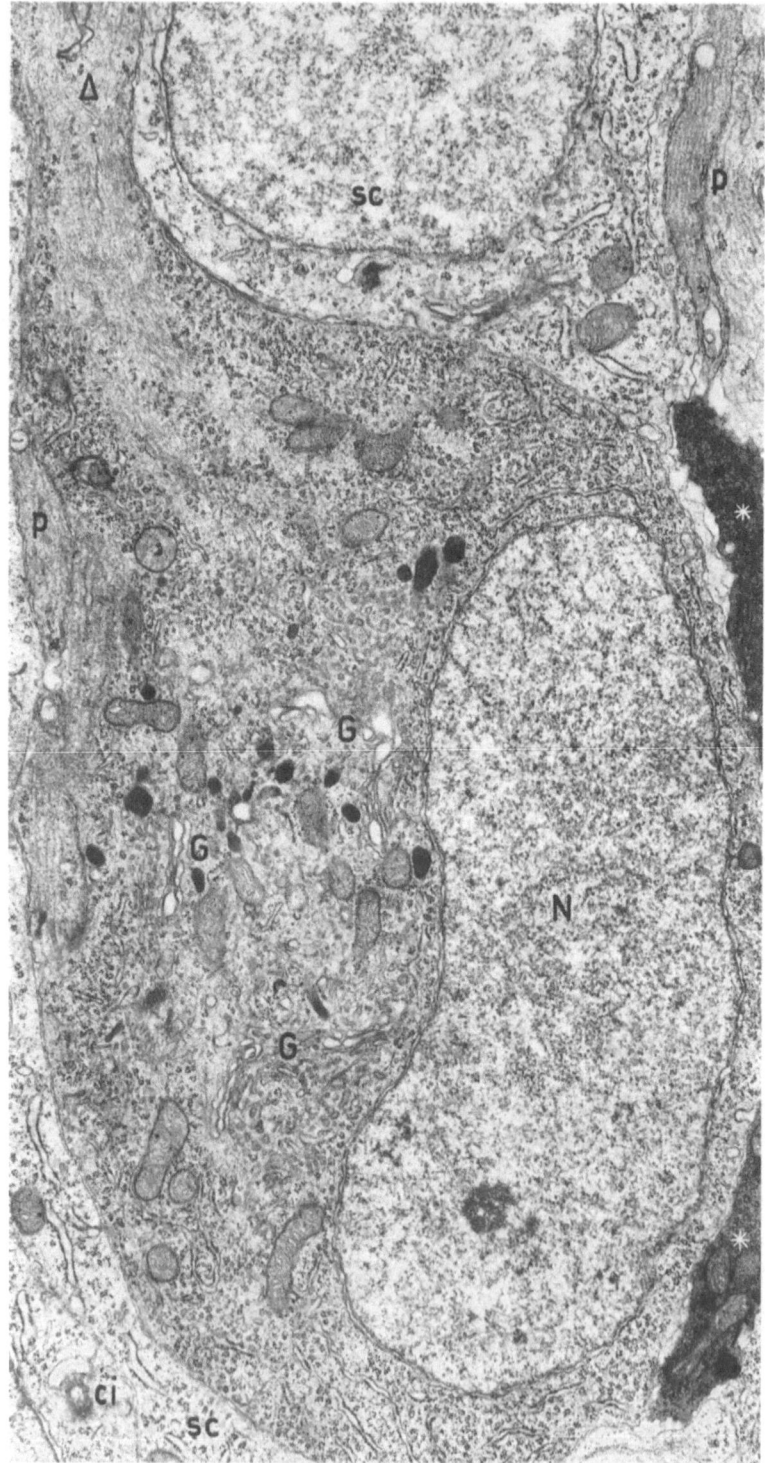

Fig. 9

neuroblast has a more highly developed Golgi complex. This lies mainly in the clearer central zone of the perikaryon (Fig. 9). More than one section of the Golgi complex is always evident in each section passing through the central zone of the perikaryon; each section of the Golgi complex consists of 4–5 long cisternae and many vesicles. During the transformation of the primitive neuroblast into the intermediate neuroblast, the Golgi complex undergoes therefore both an enlargement and a change in position.

In the pseudo-unipolar nerve cells the Golgi complex does not show a definite localization; its sections seem distributed at random throughout the perikaryon (Fig. 21). Sometimes the smooth-surfaced areas of the endoplasmic reticulum membranes adjacent to the Golgi complex exhibit small blebs, whose diameter is the same as that of the small vesicles of the Golgi complex. Such patterns recall those observed by Zeigel and Dalton (1962) in protein-secreting cells.

c) Centrioles and Cilia. Centrioles (Figs. 6c, 8) and isolated cilia are sometimes observed in sections of cells of the neuroblastic line. Usually one pair of centrioles is present in each cell; one of the two centrioles in the pair serves as the basal body of the cilium.

In the transitional elements between the undifferentiated cell and the primitive neuroblast these organelles do not show a fixed position. In the primitive neuroblast, instead, centrioles (Fig. 6c) and cilium lie in one of the cones of cytoplasm, often near the nucleus. A Golgi complex is usually evident in the vicinity of the centrioles (Fig. 6c). In the intermediate neuroblast, centrioles and cilium lie in the clearer central zone of the perikaryon; the centrioles are partially surrounded by a Golgi complex.

The long axis of one centriole usually makes an angle with the long axis of the other centriole in the same pair. Each centriole appears as a cylinder 0.20 to 0.25 μ in diameter and about 0.30 μ in length; its wall contains the usual nine triplet fibers. Sometimes dense satellite bodies can be seen in the vicinity of the centrioles. Each cilium projects into a channel formed by a deep invagination of the plasma membrane. The ciliary shaft measures from about 0.20 μ to about 0.25 μ in diameter and lacks fibers or tubular structures in its central portion.

d) Mitochondria. During the transformation of the undifferentiated cell into a neuroblast, a striking increase in the chondriome takes place. In fact, counts of the mitochondrial profiles in the spinal ganglia of the chick embryo have shown that the average number of mitochondrial profiles per perikaryal section passing through the nucleus (Fig. 11) is 1.4 in the undifferentiated cells, and 15 in the primitive neuroblasts (Pannese, 1966b).

Fig. 9. Intermediate neuroblast (spinal ganglion of a chick embryo: 18000 ×). The nucleus (*N*) is eccentric and concave on the surface facing the central zone of the perikaryon. In the perikaryon two regions can be distinguished. The peripheral region contains chiefly rough-surfaced cisternae of the endoplasmic reticulum and free ribosomal clusters. The central zone contains chiefly Golgi complexes (*G*), mitochondria, dense bodies, etc. Only one (△) of the two cell processes is evident in this section, the other arising from the perikaryon at another level. * indicates a degenerating cell. *ci* cilium in a satellite cell (sc); *p* processes which belong to other neuroblasts

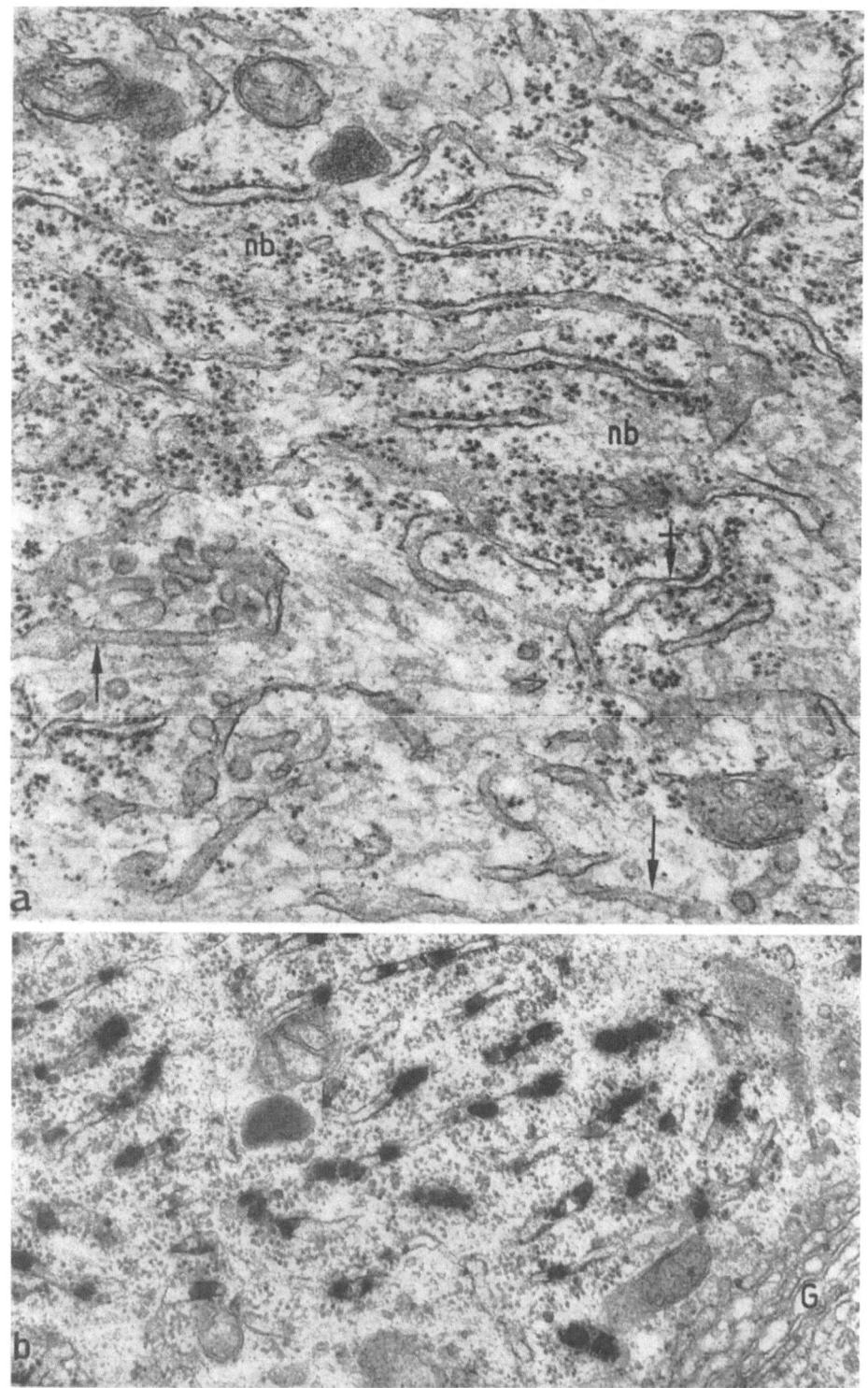

Fig. 10 a and b

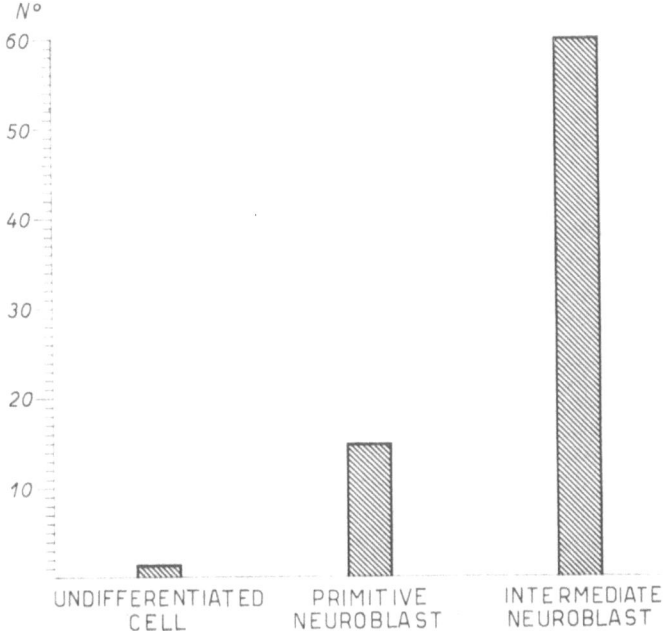

Fig. 11. Histogram showing the average number (N, on the ordinate) of mitochondrial profiles per perikaryal section passing through the nucleus respectively in the undifferentiated cell, in the primitive neuroblast, and in the intermediate neuroblast of the chick embryo spinal ganglia

The chondriome is even more abundant in the intermediate neuroblast, where the mitochondria lie mainly in the clearer central zone of the perikaryon: in these cells (Fig. 11), in fact, the average number of mitochondrial profiles per perikaryal section passing through the nucleus is 60 (Pannese, 1966b). Although the values reported above are merely indicative, they are sufficient to picture the tremendous mitochondrial increase, which takes place during differentiation and maturation of the ganglionic neuroblast.

Many neuroblasts undergo differentiation in the lateroventral region of spinal ganglia in chick embryos during the 4th and 5th incubation day. In the same period and in the same region of spinal ganglia the structures listed below were

Fig. 10a and b. Endoplasmic reticulum in mature nerve cells. Fig. a (spinal ganglion of an adult rabbit: 60000×) shows a perikaryal portion of a mature neuron. A Nissl body (nb), consisting of a stack of rough-surfaced cisternae, and of free ribosomal clusters, is evident in the upper half of the figure. Microtubules, neurofilaments, and smooth-surfaced profiles (some of which are arrowed) of the endoplasmic reticulum can be seen especially in the lower half of the figure. A point of continuity between a rough-surfaced and a smooth-surfaced portion of a cisterna is marked by a crossed arrow. Fig. b (spinal ganglion of an adult fowl, Karnovsky's method for AChE activity: 30000×; preparation by E. Pannese, L. Luciano, S. Iurato, and E. Reale) shows a Nissl body in the perikaryon of a mature neuron. The granules of the reaction product appear localized within the rough-surfaced cisternae. In the lower right is a part of a Golgi complex (G) whose cisternae do not contain reaction product

steadily observed (Pannese, 1966a, b), whichever fixative was used (OsO_4, glutaraldehyde, or $KMnO_4$). As it will be seen on p. 37 to 39, these structures could be in some way related to the quantitative increase in the chondriome.

α) Membranous whorls continuous with the nuclear envelope. The membranes of these whorls are clearly in continuity with the outer nuclear membrane while the inner nuclear membrane does not seem to be interrupted at the level of the membranous whorls, and it separates the latter from the nucleoplasm. These whorls may reach the maximum dimensions (measured on series of sections containing the whole whorl) of $0.5 \times 0.7 \times 1$ μ.

While many ribosomes are attached to the cytoplasmic surface of the outer nuclear membrane, which is therefore rough-surfaced, the membranes of the whorls are usually smooth-surfaced. A variable amount of free granules is found in general in the spaces intervening between the membranes of each whorl.

β) Membranous whorls showing a finely granular material of medium density in their more peripheral portion. In section, this granular material often appears crescent-shaped and bounded by an envelope consisting of two membranes. Some membranous whorls enclosing a crescent of granular material are continuous with the nuclear envelope; others lack any apparent continuity, although they lie often in close proximity to the nuclear envelope.

γ) Membranous whorls continuous with mitochondria. These whorls show the same features as those described under α), but their membranes are clearly in continuity with the membranes of the envelope and cristae of mitochondria. Serial micrographs reveal that the whorls consisting of many membranous turns are, as a rule, in continuity with small mitochondria, while whorls consisting of a few turns are in general continuous with large mitochondria. The latter organelles are not only large in size, but also irregular in shape.

Moreover, in series of sections a membranous whorl in continuity both with the outer nuclear membrane and with a mitochondrion has occasionally been observed. The continuity of the whorl with the nuclear membrane is usually evident only in some sections of the series, and the continuity of the whorl with the mitochondrion only in other sections of the same series.

It should be emphasized that the outer nuclear membrane, the membranes of the whorls described above, and the mitochondrial membranes have the same mean thickness.

e) Microtubules and Filaments. In the transitional elements between the undifferentiated cell and the primitive neuroblast both microtubules and filaments are present. The microtubules may appear as scattered individual profiles (Fig. 15b), or associated in fine bundles in the peripheral region of the cell; the filaments (Fig. 5) appear usually as individual profiles, more rarely associated in fine bundles.

In the primitive neuroblast and in the successive cells of the neuroblastic line, the filaments may be called neurofilaments. In sections through the major axis of the primitive neuroblast a bundle of closely packed filaments with a wavy course can sometimes be seen (Fig. 6a, b). From the site of emergence of a process this bundle arrives near the nucleus. This bundle of filaments probably corresponds to the neurofibril described by Besta (1904a) in the same position of neuroblasts (Fig. 3b) with the Cajal's method (see p. 15). The cytoplasmic area occupied by this bundle of filaments is devoid of other organelles, and so it appears lighter than the remaining perikaryon, which contains many free and membrane-attached ribosomes (Fig. 6b). In other sections of the same cell other neurofilaments and microtubules appear individually scattered in the perikaryon.

In the intermediate neuroblast (Fig. 9), microtubules and neurofilaments are very numerous, particularly in the clearer central zone of the perikaryon, where they appear interspersed among other organelles (mitochondria, dense bodies, Golgi complex, etc.). The microtubules are usually scattered as individual units, while the neurofilaments are arranged in fine bundles. In some sections, microtubules and neurofilaments can be seen funneling into the bases of the processes from the clearer central zone of the perikaryon. Sometimes a small bundle of neurofilaments is observed, confined in the peripheral portion of the perikaryon which intervenes between the sites of emergence of the processes. Such bundle probably corresponds to the arched fibrillar bundle described by Cajal (1904) (see p. 15).

A quantitative evaluation of so thin structures is not easy: it can be maintained, however, that in comparison with the primitive neuroblast the intermediate neuroblast contains a larger number of microtubules and neurofilaments in the perikaryon. During neuroblastic maturation, microtubules and neurofilaments increase, therefore, in number in the perikaryon.

In the pseudo-unipolar nerve cells (Figs. 10a, 21) microtubules and neurofilaments appear throughout the perikaryon. Neurofilaments are much more numerous than microtubules; the former are usually loosely aggregated in small bundles, while the latter appear as individual units. The bundles of neurofilaments and the microtubules lie in the space free of other cytoplasmic organelles (Nissl bodies, mitochondria, dense bodies, Golgi complex, etc.). From the perikaryon microtubules and neurofilaments funnel into the basis of the process.

2. Nucleus

Up to now, the structural changes which take place in the nucleus during neuronal differentiation have received little attention. To my knowledge systematic studies at the electron microscope level of the nuclear changes occurring during the development of the spinal ganglia nerve cells are wanting. These changes were recently studied in the developing Purkinje cells by Radouco-Thomas et al. (1971); their findings can be summarized as follows.

The chromatin appears condensed in the undifferentiated cell nucleus, then it undergoes a dispersion in the early neuroblast and finally it becomes homogeneously distributed in the intermediate neuroblast. The nucleolus appears as a compact structure in the undifferentiated cell and in the early neuroblast, then it undergoes a segregation-like process, thus acquiring in the intermediate neuroblast the network structure of the adult neuron.

3. Processes

Structural differences between peripheral and central processes of the neuroblasts were described in the spinal ganglia of the chick embryo (Barasa et al., 1970). In particular the proportion of microtubules to neurofilaments differs in the two opposite processes (Fig. 6d, e), microtubules being more numerous than neurofilaments in the peripheral process, while the opposite occurs in the central process.

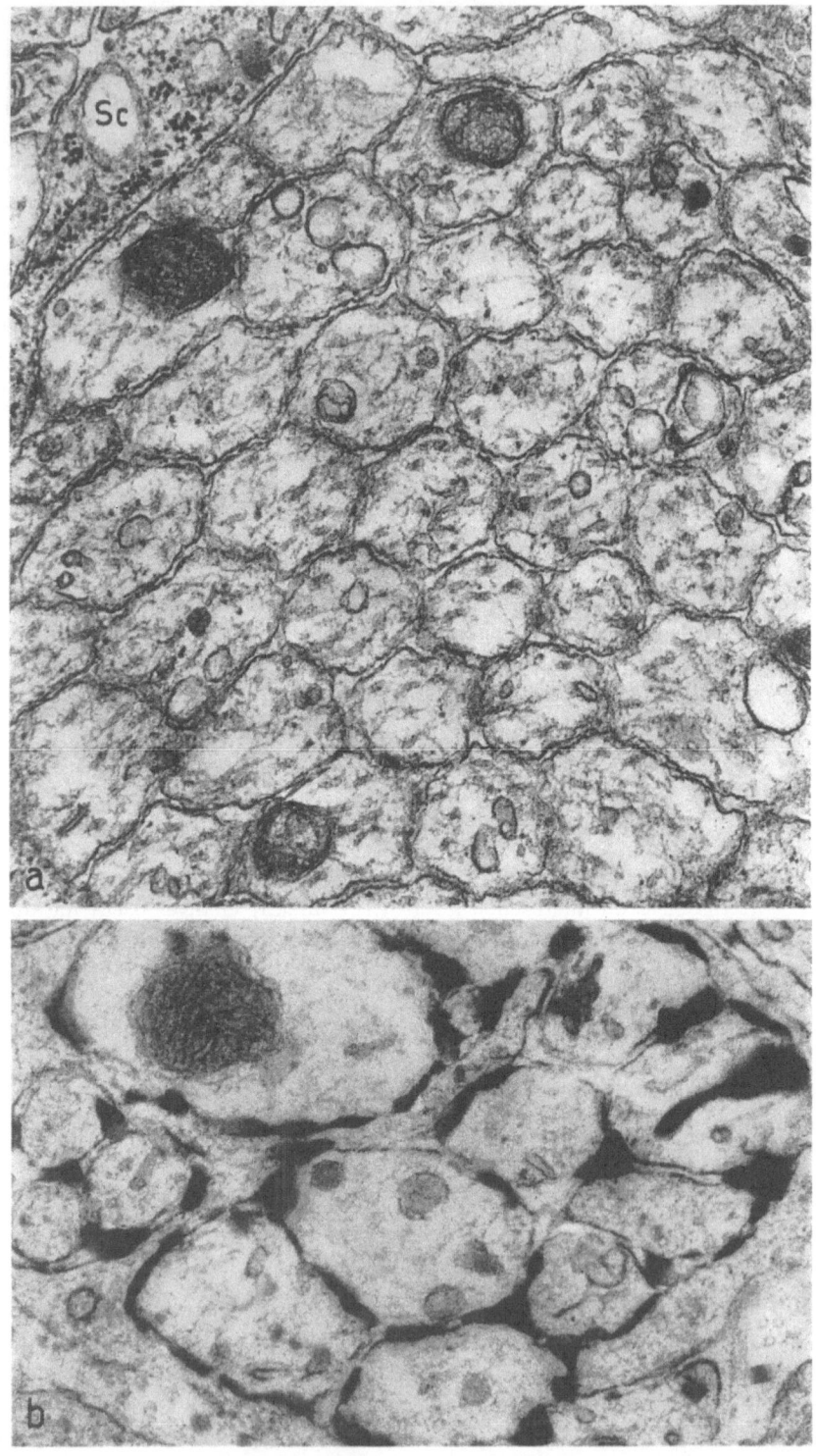

Fig. 12a and b

The central process of the neuroblast of the spinal ganglia (Figs. 6d, 12a) contains microtubules (230–250 Å in diameter), neurofilaments (90–110 Å in thickness), free ribosomes, profiles of the smooth-surfaced endoplasmic reticulum, smooth-surfaced vesicles and mitochondria (Tennyson, 1965, 1970a; Yamada et al., 1971). Microtubules and neurofilaments are arranged parallel to the long axis of the process. The microtubules are not arranged in fascicles in the initial segment of the central process (Tennyson, 1970a). This fasciculation of the microtubules is also lacking in the adult nerve cells of the spinal ganglia, while it is evident in adult multipolar nerve cells (Palay et al., 1968; Peters et al., 1968; Westrum, 1970). Pinocytotic vesicles occur along the plasma membrane of the processes of the spinal ganglia neuroblasts (Fig. 6d).

It may be recalled here, that free ribosomes were also found in myelinated axons of neurons of the spinal ganglia of adult rats (Zelená, 1970, 1972) and in both the embryonic and fetal axons (Lyser, 1964, 1968a; Caley and Maxwell, 1968), in the initial segment of adult nerve cells (Palay et al., 1968; Peters et al., 1968; Jones and Powell, 1969; Westrum, 1970), in an axon beyond the initial segment of an adult nerve cell (Peters, 1971) from other regions of the nervous system. Membrane-attached ribosomes were found in the initial segment of the axon of adult cat motoneurons (Conradi, 1966). It should be remembered here, however, that the axons described by Jones and Powell (1969) have been interpreted as dendrites by Famiglietti and Peters (1972).

Passing from an early to a later developmental stage some structural changes are observed in the central process. In later developmental stages the central process generally contains many more neurofilaments (Fig. 9) than in the earlier period (Tennyson, 1970a, in rabbit embryos).

The growth cone of the central process of the spinal ganglia neuroblasts of the rabbit was studied in vivo by Tennyson (1970a). At an early developmental stage, the growth cone appears under the electron microscope as a bulbous varicosity (6 to 13 μ in length and 2 to 5 μ in width) from which thin membranous extensions sprout. This varicosity contains irregularly shaped vesicles, 450 to 700 Å in diameter, and a few mitochondria embedded in a finely filamentous matrix; the thin membranous extensions contain only a finely filamentous matrix. At a later developmental stage, the growth cone of the central process contains a greater amount and variety of organelles than in earlier stages: namely, smooth-surfaced cisternae of the endoplasmic reticulum, mitochondria, dense bodies, clusters of ribosomes and scattered microtubules and neurofilaments (Fig. 13). At this stage the structure of the growth cone of the central process of the spinal ganglia neuroblast resembles that of the cones of cultured sympathetic neuroblasts

Fig. 12a and b. Processes of ganglionic neuroblasts. Fig. a (spinal ganglion of a chick embryo: 50000 ×) shows central processes in a cross section. Each process contains microtubules, and neurofilaments; some show also profiles of the smooth-surfaced endoplasmic reticulum, and mitochondria. At this stage of development many processes are still grouped into bundles surrounded by a common Schwann cell sheath (Sc). Fig. b (spinal ganglion of a chick embryo, Karnovsky's method for AChE activity: 60000 ×; preparation by E. Pannese, L. Luciano, S. Iurato, and E. Reale) shows several processes in a cross section. Granules of the reaction product are evident in the clefts between the processes

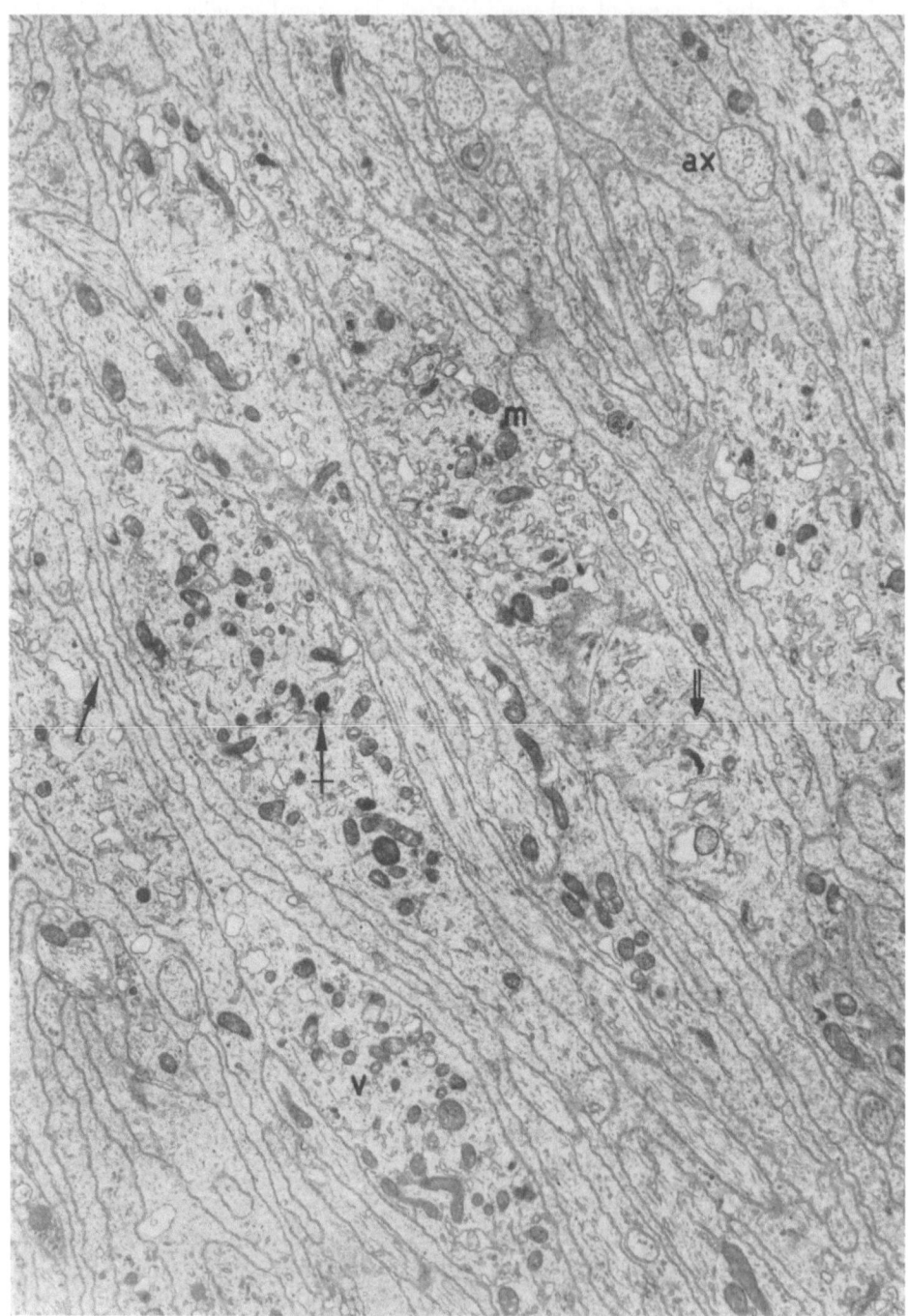

Fig. 13. Transverse section of the junction of growth cones of the dorsal root with the posterior fasciculus (rabbit fetus: 9300 ×). Thin filopodial processes (arrow) filled with a finely filamentous matrix material, extend from bulbous varicosities (*v*), containing mitochondria (*m*), dense bodies (crossed arrow), profiles of the smooth-surfaced endoplasmic reticulum (double arrow), vesicles, and filaments. Axons (*ax*) of the posterior fasciculus are cut in cross section. (Courtesy of Dr. Tennyson)

(Bunge, 1973) and that of the cones of regenerating nerve fibers (Estable *et al.*, 1957; Wechsler and Hager, 1961; Wettstein and Sotelo, 1963; Lampert, 1967; Lentz, 1967).

The growth cone of the processes of the spinal ganglia neuroblasts in the chick embryo was studied in tissue cultures by Yamada *et al.* (1971). The growth cone appears as an enlargement at the tip of the elongating process, from which long, thin microspikes and thin membranes extend outward. The growth cone contains large amount of smooth-surfaced endoplasmic reticulum, vesicles, neurofilaments (100 Å in thickness), a few microtubules, and a peripheral network of filaments (40–60 Å in thickness), extending into the microspikes.

Also growth cones of neurites from other regions of the nervous system were studied with the electron microscope (Bodian, 1966, 1968; del Cerro and Snider, 1968; Kawana *et al.*, 1971). The structure of these growth cones differs a little from that of the above mentioned cones. Such discrepancies might depend on the location of the cones in the nervous system, on the influence of the different techniques applied on these very delicate structures, or finally on the fact that the cones are highly dynamic entities, whose structure may change under different conditions.

Microspikes identical in shape and structure to those protruding from growth cones, also extend laterally from the processes of the spinal ganglia neuroblasts cultured *in vitro* (Yamada *et al.*, 1971).

C. Hypotheses on the Mechanisms of Organellogenesis and Functional Considerations

We shall now briefly deal with the possible mechanisms by which the events characterizing neuronal differentiation take place and with the functional meaning of some cytoplasmic organelles. Some of the mechanisms of organellogenesis which will be discussed in this section do not only deal with the neuroblast but are of a more general interest.

a) The various views held on the mechanisms of the *biogenesis of the membranes of the endoplasmic reticulum* can be summarized as follows.

α) The membranes of the endoplasmic reticulum are synthesized *de novo* in the hyaloplasm (Fawcett, 1955; Ferreira, 1959; Rouiller and Simon, 1962; Cossel, 1964; Whaley *et al.*, 1964) through the following steps: formation of small smooth-surfaced vesicles and tubules, attachment of ribosomes to the membranes, and, finally, coalescence of the vesicles and tubules to form large cisternae.

β) The Golgi complex takes part in the formation of the endoplasmic reticulum membranes by giving rise to smooth-surfaced vesicles, which become rough-surfaced cisternae through attachment of ribosomes, and by undergoing expansion or coalescence (Hay, 1958, in the amphibian cartilage; Wohlfarth-Bottermann and Moericke, 1959, in the salivary glands of Invertebrates; Tennyson, 1965, in neuroblasts of the rabbit embryo; Stäubli *et al.*, 1966, in the midgut epithelial cells of mosquitoes).

γ) The membranes of the endoplasmic reticulum arise from the nuclear envelope (Gay, 1956; Moses, 1956; Miller, 1958; Parks, 1962; Behnke and Moe, 1964; Kessel, 1964; Dvořák, 1968; Pannese, 1968a; Wenzel *et al.*, 1973). Also according to Porter (1961), the nuclear envelope could be the source of the newly formed cisternae of the endoplasmic reticulum.

δ) The endoplasmic reticulum membranes originate through a double mechanism: by expansion of the nuclear envelope and by *de novo* synthesis in the hyaloplasm (Wechsler, 1965, in the chick embryo neuroblasts), or from the Golgi complex and, to a lesser degree, from the nuclear envelope (Meller *et al.*, 1966, in the chick embryo neuroblasts).

Obviously, a dynamic sequence of events may hardly be reconstructed from fixed preparations; the electron microscope images may however offer some indications as to the biogenesis of the endoplasmic reticulum in developing nerve cells of the spinal ganglia. As mentioned on p. 16, when the primitive neuroblasts at an early developmental stage undergo a striking increase of the rough-surfaced endoplasmic reticulum, they do not contain numerous, small, isolated units of this reticulum but a three-dimensional system of long interconnected cisternae (Fig. 7a, b). These findings do not agree with the hypotheses listed under α and β. The hypothesis listed under β seems improbable also on the basis of the general knowledge now available on the synthesis of the membrane components. Also the close relationship between a rough-surfaced cisterna and smooth-surfaced cisternae of the Golgi complex (Fig. 6c) does not seem very significant as regards endoplasmic reticulum biogenesis. This relationship could be merely accidental, or might be related to the transfer of enzymes from the rough-surfaced endoplasmic reticulum to the Golgi complex (Kessel, 1971), as well as to the morphogenesis and/or enlargement of the Golgi complex.

The rough-surfaced cisternae appear sometimes continuous with the nuclear envelope mainly in the primitive neuroblasts (Fig. 7a, b); this finding seems to agree with the hypothesis on the formation of the rough-surfaced endoplasmic reticulum from the nuclear envelope. Of course, the physical continuity is not sufficient by itself to prove that endoplasmic reticulum membranes take their origin from the nuclear envelope; in fact, the continuity could be established soon after the endoplasmic reticulum has appeared. It must be stressed, however, that, as many examples demonstrate, the nuclear envelope of embryonic cells is capable of remarkable expansive growth, i.e. of membrane production (see, e.g., Kessel, 1964, 1971; Pannese, 1966c). Taking into consideration both the finding of rough-surfaced cisternae in continuity with the nuclear envelope in primitive neuroblasts and the ability of the nuclear envelope to produce membrane, the hypothesis listed under γ), i.e. formation of the rough-surfaced endoplasmic reticulum from the nuclear envelope, appears the most probable during neuroblastic differentiation in the spinal ganglia.

As stated above, in comparison with the primitive neuroblasts (Fig. 6a), the intermediate neuroblasts (Fig. 9) and the pseudo-unipolar nerve cells (Fig. 21) have a more highly developed and organized rough-surfaced endoplasmic reticulum.

The continuity between the rough-surfaced endoplasmic reticulum and the nuclear envelope has been seldom observed in the intermediate neuroblasts and it has never been detected in the pseudo-unipolar nerve cells. On this basis, it could be supposed that in the intermediate neuroblasts and in the pseudo-unipolar nerve cells the rough-surfaced endoplasmic reticulum increases in volume through an intrinsic expansive growth of its membranes.

If the rough-surfaced endoplasmic reticulum of the primitive neuroblast actually takes origin from the nuclear envelope, the nuclear envelope could be regarded as a sort of matrix which by its expansive growth might supply the neuroblast with the first significant amount of rough-surfaced endoplasmic reticulum. Afterwards, the rough-surfaced endoplasmic reticulum of the neuroblast might increase in volume through an intrinsic expansive growth.

As far as the smooth-surfaced endoplasmic reticulum is concerned, the fact that (a) this organelle appears in the neuroblasts when the rough-surfaced endoplasmic reticulum is well developed, and that (b) smooth-surfaced cisternae often appear in continuity with the rough-surfaced cisternae, may suggest that the smooth-surfaced endoplasmic reticulum may arise from the rough-surfaced endoplasmic reticulum. Such an origin has been suggested for the smooth-surfaced endoplasmic reticulum of the rat hepatocyte by Dallner et al. (1966) and by Orrenius and Ericsson (1966).

b) That enlargement of the Golgi complex may take place by growth and division of this organelle was suggested long ago on the basis of light microscopy studies (see Gatenby, 1919). This hypothesis has been more recently reproposed on the basis of electron microscopy studies (Afzelius, 1956; Grassé, 1957; Gatenby, 1960; Carasso and Favard, 1961; Dalton, 1961; Wischnitzer, 1962; Buvat, 1963; Clowes and Juniper, 1964; Yamamoto and Onozato, 1965; Mollenhauer and Morré, 1966; Whaley, 1966; Ward and Ward, 1968; Kiermayer, 1970). According to other authors, however, the Golgi complex could enlarge by receiving membrane from other cell structures. In particular, the plasma membrane (Daniels, 1964), the endoplasmic reticulum (Grimstone, 1959; Essner and Novikoff, 1962; Kessel, 1968; Flickinger, 1969; Hollande, 1970; Morré et al., 1971; Wise, 1972) and the nuclear envelope (Ackerman, 1962; Moore and McAlear, 1963; Bouck, 1965; Caley and Maxwell, 1968; Falk and Kleinig, 1968; Fawcett and McNutt, 1969; Longo and Anderson, 1969; Scharrer and Wurzelmann, 1969a; Stang-Voss, 1970; Chrétien, 1971; Kessel, 1971; Ovtracht, 1971; Dubois, 1972; Weston et al., 1972) have been considered potential sources of membrane which can be incorporated into the Golgi complex. The origin of the Golgi complex from lamellar bodies formed within the nucleus has been suggested by Ruby and Webster (1972).

To my knowledge, no evidence has been found either of a division of the Golgi complex, or of an intervention of the plasma membrane in the enlargement of the Golgi complex during neuronal differentiation in the spinal ganglia.

Regarding the possible role of the rough-surfaced endoplasmic reticulum, it was already mentioned (see p. 23) that in the primitive neuroblasts, rough-surfaced profiles may be found in proximity to the smooth-surfaced cisternae of the Golgi complex (Fig. 6c). As pointed out previously (see p. 34), this relationship could be merely accidental, or it might be related to the transfer of enzymes from the rough-surfaced endoplasmic reticulum to the Golgi-complex, or to the morphogenesis and/or enlargement of the Golgi complex.

Also the nuclear envelope may show peculiar relationships with the Golgi complex (Fig. 7d) in the primitive neuroblasts (see p. 23). Such relationships could indicate that the nuclear envelope is involved in the production of membrane destined to be incorporated into the Golgi complex, and this view may appear warranted when considering that the nuclear envelope of the embryonic cells has apparently a remarkable ability for membrane production. The nuclear envelope and the rough-surfaced endoplasmic reticulum appear, therefore, as the main cell structures involved in the morphogenesis of the Golgi complex. On account of the finding that in the intermediate neuroblasts and in the pseudo-unipolar nerve cells the relationships between the nuclear envelope and the Golgi complex are no longer apparent, while the relationships between the rough-surfaced endoplasmic reticulum and the Golgi complex are still evident, it may be supposed that in these cells the Golgi complex is maintained and/or enlarged by membrane coming from the rough-surfaced endoplasmic reticulum. Such dynamic relationships between the rough-surfaced endoplasmic reticulum and the Golgi complex probably occur also in other kinds of cells (see, e.g., Zeigel and Dalton, 1962).

c) In the spinal ganglion of the chick embryo the average number of mito-chondrial profiles (Fig. 11) in the primitive neuroblast is about 10 times greater than in the undifferentiated cell (see p. 25). Therefore, a conspicuous *increase in the chondriome* takes place during neuroblastic differentiation.

The formation of new mitochondria is probably a general process. First of all, it is well known that new mitochondria can be formed in the cells which divide repeatedly, in cells in which massive mitochondrial degeneration takes place, and in the cells which increase considerably in size: thereby the mitochondrial density of these cells could be maintained constant. Moreover, formation of new mitochondria does occur not only in the cell classes mentioned but probably also in many other cell classes for the renewal of the mitochondrial population: in fact, the turnover time of a mitochondrion might be quite short, e.g., about 5–10 days in the adult mammalian liver (Fletcher and Sanadi, 1961). Contrasting opinions have been held, however, on the mechanism of mitochondrial forma-tion. The chief mechanisms which have been proposed hitherto can be briefly summarized as follows.

α) Formation through division of pre-existing mitochondria. This hypothesis rests chiefly on the following observations. In living cells cultured *in vitro* images of mitochondria which seem to divide have frequently been observed (Lewis and Lewis, 1915; Chèvremont, 1953; Frederic, 1958). Centrally attenuated mitochondria have often been recorded with the electron microscope and inter-preted as mitochondria undergoing division (Fawcett, 1955; Tahmisian *et al.*, 1956; Wohlfarth-Bottermann, 1957; Lund *et al.*, 1958; Karasaki, 1959; André, 1962; Bahr and Zeitler, 1962; von Maltzahn and Mühlethaler, 1962; Elliot and Bak, 1964; Lafontaine and Allard, 1964; Diers, 1966; Hawley and Wagner, 1967; Tandler *et al.*, 1969). Also quantitative radioautographic studies on *Neurospora crassa* labelled with radioactive choline (Luck, 1963, 1965), have supplied evidence consistent with the formation of new mitochondria through division of pre-existing ones.

β) Formation from microbodies (Rouiller and Bernhard, 1956; Roth, 1957; Belt, 1958; Weissenfels, 1958; Ferreira, 1959; Oberling, 1959; Hudson and Hart-mann, 1961). This mechanism, however, is considered unlikely by Essner and Novikoff (1960, 1961).

γ) Formation from other membranous structures pre-existing in the cell. Nearly all the membranous structures of the cell have been called upon as possible sources of mitochondria: the membranes of the Golgi complex (Lever, 1956;

Berger, 1964), the membranes of the endoplasmic reticulum (Buvat, 1959; Bade, 1964), some small cytoplasmic vesicles (Wohlfarth-Bottermann, 1957) and smooth vacuoles (Threadgold and Lasker, 1967; Norberg, 1972), the plasma membrane (Geren and Schmitt, 1954; Robertson, 1959; De Robertis and Bleichmar, 1962; Schjeide and McCandless, 1962; Stroganova and Monakhova, 1965), the pino-cytotic vesicles (Gey et al., 1955), the cytoplasmic membranes of yeasts (Linnane et al., 1962; Wallace and Linnane, 1964), and the nuclear envelope (Hoffman and Grigg, 1958; Brandt and Pappas, 1959; Bell and Mühlethaler, 1964; Pannese, 1966a, b; Stang-Voss and Staubesand, 1970).

δ) Genesis by *de novo* synthesis. This hypothesis was first formulated by Beckwith (1914) and often reproposed (see Newcomer, 1940 for a review); more recently it was advanced again by Harvey (1946) who studied centrifuged eggs by light microscopy. However, Harvey's conclusions are not consistent with the electron microscopical findings on centrifuged eggs (Lansing et al., 1952; Pasteels et al., 1959; Berg and Humphreys, 1960; Gross et al., 1960). The hypothesis mentioned has recently been reproposed by Zollinger (1956), and Berger (1964).

ε) According to other hypotheses, in oocytes the mitochondria would be formed from yolk granules (Lanzavecchia and Le Coultre, 1958), or in relation with a dense material which passes from the nucleus into the cytoplasm (Balinsky and Devis, 1963; Lanzavecchia and Mangioni, 1963; Schjeide et al., 1964). In oocytes materials coming from the nucleus could be incorporated into the matrix of differentiating mitochondria (Scharrer and Wurzelmann, 1969b). In enterocytes of embryonic chick the mitochondria have been said to develop from lipid droplets (Holman, 1969). In some liver cells new mitochondria would form inside pre-existing ones (David, 1962).

As among the various views on mitochondrial formation some at least are founded on reliable observations, it seems possible that there may be indeed different mechanisms of mitochondrial formation which operate in different cells or in a given cell under different conditions, or at different stages in the develop-ment. All these mechanisms could lead to the formation of the mitochondrial supporting structure; the synthesis of the specific mitochondrial enzymes would be the only process common to all the mechanisms of mitochondrial formation hypothesized so far. The latter process could be the only truly specific one.

The increase in the chondriome which takes place during the differentiation of the primitive neuroblast is quite conspicuous, and rapid; one would expect, therefore, that a careful study by electron microscopy may reveal images related to the increase in the chondriome. In the cells undergoing neuroblastic differentia-tion, however, only a negligible number of mitochondria show constrictions of their contour; it seems unlikely, therefore, that in these cells the chondriome may increase by growth and division of pre-existing mitochondria. Moreover, images interpretable as related to other mechanisms of mitochondrial formation have not been observed. Hence, the hypothesis has been advanced that the structures described on p. 27 and 28 may actually be related to formation of mitochondria. The following mechanism (Fig. 14) has been proposed (Pannese, 1966a, b).

The outer nuclear membrane undergoes expansion in a limited area and folds up, thus forming a number of turns; this membranous whorl consists at the beginning of a few, loosely arranged membranous turns. Subsequently, the latter

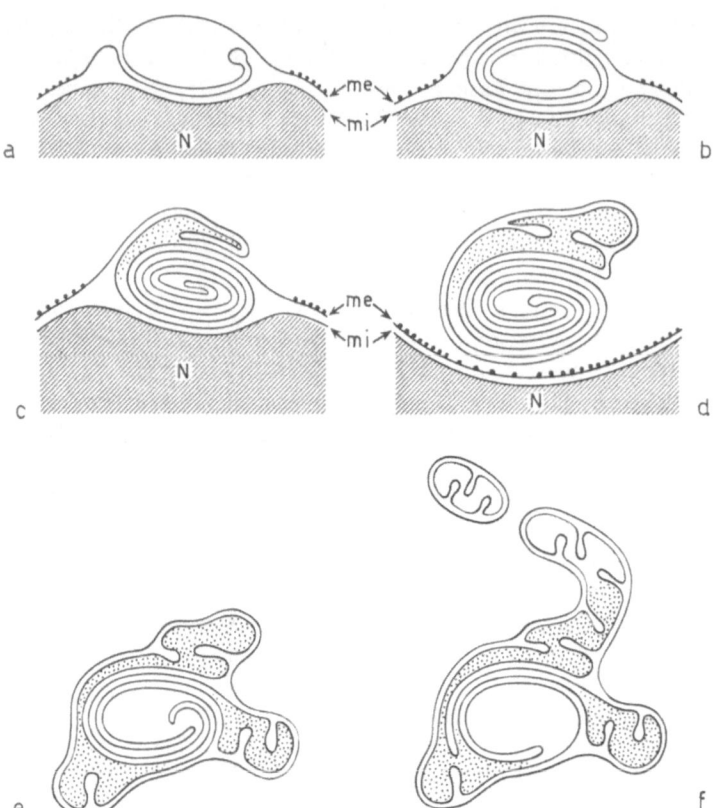

Fig. 14. Diagram showing the possible formation mechanism of new mitochondria from the nuclear envelope in the ganglionic neuroblasts. *me* outer nuclear membrane, *mi* inner nuclear membrane, *N* nucleus. [From E. Pannese: Z. Zellforsch. **72**, 295–324 (1966)]

increase in number and become tightly packed. In the course of the formation of the membranous whorl, a number of granules remain trapped within the membranous turns of the whorl. Later on, a granular material appears in the peripheral portion of the membranous whorl; this material could be the precursor of the mitochondrial matrix. When the granular material commences to form, the whorl may still be continuous with the nuclear envelope, or it may lie free in the hyaloplasm. While the granular material increases in amount, the membranous whorl gradually unrolls. The granular material becomes the mitochondrial matrix, and the membranous whorl gives rise to the mitochondrial membranes. At this stage, structures are found which consist of a membranous whorl and of a portion which shows already the morphological features of a mitochondrion. The whorl proper seems to undergo reduction in parallel to the gradual increase of the mitochondrial portion. These structures lie usually free in the cytoplasmic matrix; sometimes, however, one of these formations may be found which still retains its continuity with the outer nuclear membrane. From a membranous whorl, a mitochondrion may thus be formed.

This hypothesis appears compatible with the results of the measurements of the thickness of the outer nuclear membrane, of the membranes of the whorls, and of the mitochondrial membranes: in the differentiating neuron of the spinal ganglion all these membranes are practically identical in thickness. Also in other kinds of cells an equal thickness of the mitochondrial membranes and of the membranes of the nuclear envelope was reported (Yamamoto, 1963).

The mechanism of mitochondrial formation hypothesized here, is reminiscent in some stages of the one suggested by Bell and Mühlethaler (1964) to explain mitochondrial formation in the egg cells of a fern.

Sometimes in the spinal ganglia of the chick embryo membranous whorls can be found in the extracellular space. These whorls, which arise from the nuclear envelope, could be regarded as the result of abortive events occurring in the course of mitochondrial formation.

In connection with the account given on p. 37 and 38, it could be assumed that during neuroblastic differentiation the early mitochondria can be formed from the nuclear envelope. The formation of mitochondria from the nuclear envelope could involve the transfer of nuclear genetic information essential for the subsequent increase in the chondriome, which could well take place by a different mechanism (e.g., by growth and division of the mitochondria).

d) *Microtubules* are evident both in the undifferentiated cells (Fig. 2a) and in the transitional elements (Fig. 15b) between the undifferentiated cells and the primitive neuroblasts. As both these types of cell divide by mitosis, it is difficult to decide whether the microtubules inside these cells have been *de novo* synthesized, or are the remnants of the spindle from an earlier mitosis.

In the primitive neuroblasts the microtubules are never very numerous within the perikaryon, while they are abundant in the cell processes (Figs. 4, 6d, e). On the basis of present knowledge, a number of functions have been postulated for microtubules. It seems reasonable to believe that at least some of these hypotheses can also be applied to microtubules contained in the cell processes of the neuroblasts.

The microtubules could represent a cytoskeleton which gives support for the anisometries in cell form (Tandler and Moriber, 1966; Behnke and Zelander, 1967; Kessel, 1967; Sabnis and Jacobs, 1967; Bouck and Brown, 1970). This role seems to be instrumental in the maintenance of the cell extensions (Tilney and Porter, 1965; Bikle *et al.*, 1966). As suggested by Porter (1966), Peters and Vaughn (1967), Lyser (1968a), and Tennyson (1970a) and some experimental studies seem to indicate (Hoffman, 1952; Yamada et al., 1970, 1971; Daniels, 1972), the microtubules might provide skeletal support for the elongating processes of the neuroblasts.

Other experimental evidence (Byers and Porter, 1964; Kessel and Eichler, 1966; Tilney *et al.*, 1966; Kessel, 1967; Tilney and Porter, 1967; Tilney and Gibbins, 1969) obtained on non-nervous cells leads to believe that the microtubules are involved not only in maintenance of the asymmetric cell form as a static cytoskeleton, but in the active elongation of the cells or of the cell extensions as well. The findings of Byers and Porter (1964) on the development of the lens cells may appear particularly relevant in this connection. However, recent experimental findings of Yamada and Wessells (1971) and of Yamada *et al.* (1971)

suggest that axon elongation is due to the activity of the growth cone and is not dependent upon a "pushing" mechanism of the microtubules. According to Yamada *et al.* (1971), the growth cone could play an essential role in axonal elongation: it would represent in fact the locomotory organelle and the site of deposition of new membrane for the elongating axon.

The microtubules have been also implicated in the intracellular transport of materials (Ledbetter and Porter, 1963; Slautterback, 1963; Bikle *et al.*, 1966; Arnold, 1967; Sabnis and Jacobs, 1967). In particular, some experimental evidence seems to suggest that in nerve cells microtubules are involved in the fast (and perhaps intermediary) transport of neuroplasmic constituents (Taylor, 1967; Schmitt, 1968; Karlsson and Sjöstrand, 1969; Kreutzberg, 1969; Dahlström, 1971; Hökfelt and Dahlström, 1971; Mayor *et al.*, 1972). Other evidence suggests, however, that not only fast transport, but also slow transport in nerve cells may depend on microtubules (Fernandez *et al.*, 1970; James *et al.*, 1970). If the microtubules are actually involved in the transport of materials inside the nerve cell, such a function could be displayed also by the microtubules contained in the processes of the spinal ganglion neuroblasts and nerve cells. A transport of materials has in fact been shown both in the spinal ganglion neuroblasts (Lasher *et al.*, 1970) and in the spinal ganglion nerve cells of adult animals (Droz and Leblond, 1963; Droz, 1967; Lasek, 1968; Turbes, 1970).

Concerning the origin of the microtubules, it was suggested that these organelles may be synthesized in the centriolar complex (De-Thé, 1964; Gonatas and Robbins, 1964; Porter, 1966). As mentioned on p. 25, centrioles are often evident in neuroblasts (Figs. 6c, 8), and a close association between some microtubules and centrioles was described both in sensory (Tennyson, 1965) and motor neuroblasts (Lyser, 1968b). However, this close association seems not sufficient by itself to demonstrate that the centriole is directly involved in the formation of the neuroblastic microtubules: microtubules formed independently of the centrioles might become associated secondarily with them.

e) As it is well known, *filaments* as individual units or arranged in groups may be found in the cytoplasm of most types of cell. The thickness of these filaments may vary from one cell type to another. The available data are still insufficient to establish whether the filaments in different cell types are chemically identical or they are built of distinct fibrous proteins.

In a variety of cells the cytoplasmic filaments have been interpreted as a cytoskeletal system (Fawcett, 1966) and/or as contractile organelles (Wohlfarth-Bottermann, 1964; Cloney, 1966; Nagai and Rebhun, 1966; Rhea, 1966; Wohlman and Allen, 1968; Tilney and Gibbins, 1969; Pollard and Ito, 1970). The functions of structural support (van Breemen, 1962) and that of movement (see Schmitt and Samson, 1968 for a review) have also been attributed to neurofilaments. In particular, neurofilaments have been tentatively considered as being involved in slow neuroplasmic flow (Schmitt, 1969). However, much doubt persists at present both on the fact that neurofilaments are actually involved in neuroplasmic transport (England *et al.*, 1973), and on the exact functional relationship between microtubules and filaments in the nerve cells. The thesis that microtubules and filaments are linked in a functional relationship has been held for other types of cells (Goldman, 1971).

As to the origin of neurofilaments, it should be recalled that the ratio of neuro-filaments to microtubules in the central process of the neuroblast increases from early to later developmental stages (see p. 31). This finding is in keeping with the suggestion advanced by Peters and Vaughn (1967) in maturing axons of the rat optic nerve according to which neurofilaments may form through breakdown of microtubules. Although this hypothesis may find support in the findings of Wisniewski *et al.* (1968), it is conflicting with the chemical and morphological differences between these two organelles (see Wuerker and Palay, 1969 for a discussion): in fact, microtubule protein and filament protein isolated from nerve axoplasm differ in molecular weight, size, electrophoretic mobility, immuno-logical specificity, and amino acid composition (Davison and Huneeus, 1970; Huneeus and Davison, 1970). It may be recalled also Lyser's (1968a) hypothesis that in neuroblasts a change could occur between microtubules and neurofilaments in the opposite direction from that postulated by Peters and Vaughn (1967).

D. RNA Content

The RNA content per spinal ganglion cell was determined in the rat by Sobkowicz *et al.* (1973). *In vivo* the RNA content increases steadily from nearly 30 pg. at the 11th day of gestation to about 1000 pg. at the 11th day after birth. Then the RNA content increases very slowly until it reaches about 1250 pg. in the adult rat. In culture the RNA content per cell increases at a much slower rate than *in vivo*.

The relationship between cell size and its RNA content was also determined in the rat spinal ganglia (Sobkowicz *et al.*, 1973). In the earlier developmental stages, a large increase in cell volume is associated with only a small increase in RNA content. The opposite occurs instead towards the end of the developmental period.

E. AChE and Other Enzymatic Activities

AChE activity was first histochemically demonstrated in the developing spinal ganglia with the light microscope (Gerebtzoff, 1959; Hamburger, 1961; Strumia and Baima-Bollone, 1964). Strumia and Baima-Bollone (1964) observed that in chick embryo spinal ganglia this enzymatic activity was present from the 4th day of incubation. On the same material it was then demonstrated with the electron microscope that AChE activity is already detectable at 3 days of incuba-tion (Pannese *et al.*, 1970, 1971) and at 9 days of gestation in the spinal ganglia of rabbit embryo (Tennyson and Brzin, 1970). The higher sensitivity of the histochemical techniques for electron microscopy explains how in the spinal ganglia the AChE activity is detectable with the electron microscope in earlier stages than with the light microscope. The use of the electron microscope does not only offer the advantage mentioned but it permits also a more precise localization of the enzymatic activities.

In the embryonic spinal ganglia some cells with the structure of the undiffe-rentiated elements show a sparse AChE activity within the perinuclear cisterna (Fig. 2b), and in mitotic cells a sparse AChE activity is often apparent within

remnants of the nuclear envelope and the rough-surfaced cisternae of the endoplasmic reticulum (Pannese *et al.*, 1970, 1971, in the chick embryo). Also the
transitional cells between the undifferentiated elements and the primitive neuroblasts show AChE activity within the perinuclear cisterna, the scarce rough-
surfaced cisternae of the endoplasmic reticulum and, sometimes, also along the
plasma membrane (Pannese *et al.*, 1970, 1971, in the chick embryo). The primitive
(Fig. 7c) and intermediate neuroblasts and the pseudo-unipolar nerve cells
(Fig. 10b) show AChE activity in the following sites: within the perinuclear cisterna
(Fig. 7c), the rough-surfaced cisternae of the endoplasmic reticulum (Figs. 7c,
10b), including the subsurface cisternae, at the smooth-surfaced vesicles and
tubules of the processes, and along the axolemma (Fig. 12b) (Pannese *et al.*, 1970,
1971; Tennyson and Brzin, 1970).

   In the Golgi complex of the mitotic cells and neuroblasts a scarce AChE
activity seems to co-exist with a non specific esterase activity (Pannese *et al.*,
1971, in the chick embryo), as it has been observed also in mature nerve cells
of the spinal ganglia (Eränkö *et al.*, 1964, in the adult rat).

   Thus during the developmental period the perikaryal sites of AChE activity
are the same in all cells of the neuroblastic line (transitional cells, primitive
and intermediate neuroblasts, and pseudo-unipolar nerve cells). However, from
the primitive neuroblast to the pseudo-unipolar nerve cell the amount of reaction
product depending on the AChE activity increases considerably in parallel
to the development of the rough-surfaced endoplasmic reticulum.

   In the spinal ganglion nerve cells AChE activity is not only present during
the developmental period, but persists also in the adult animals. The main sites
of this enzymatic activity in the spinal ganglion nerve cells of the fowl appear to
be fundamentally the same both in the embryos and in the adult animals (Pannese *et al.*, 1974). Some difference can only be noted at the level of the Golgi
complex. In fact, while in the embryonic ganglia the reaction product appears
associated only with the vesicles of the Golgi complex, in the adult animals the
AChE activity can be sometimes demonstrated only in the innermost cisternae of
the Golgi complex (Pannese *et al.*, 1974). The significance of this difference is as
yet unclear.

   As to the site of AChE production in the perikaryon, this enzymatic protein
is probably synthesized by the ribosomes attached to the membranes of the
endoplasmic reticulum both in the neuroblasts (Pannese *et al.*, 1971) and in the
mature nerve cells (Fukuda and Koelle, 1959; Lewis and Shute, 1966; Schlaepfer,
1968) of the spinal ganglia.

   In the cells of the neuroblastic line the rough-surfaced endoplasmic reticulum
does not develop to a considerable extent before AChE activity appears in it.
The synthesis of this enzymatic protein seems to begin at the level of the nuclear
envelope in cells with a poorly developed endoplasmic reticulum (e. g., cells which
are probably still undifferentiated, and transitional cells between undifferentiated
elements and primitive neuroblasts); successively, it seems to propagate from the
nuclear envelope to the rough-surfaced endoplasmic reticulum as the latter
develops and increases in volume.

   The site of synthesis of AChE localized in the neuroblastic processes of the
spinal ganglia is most uncertain as yet. Admittedly, this problem has not yet

been solved either for the adult nerve cells, or for the neuroblasts. Some experimental evidence suggests that this enzymatic protein is synthesized in the perikaryon and then transported to the axon (Lewis and Hughes, 1957; Fukuda and Koelle, 1959; Lubińska et al., 1963, 1964; Eränkö and Härkönen, 1965; Kása, 1968; Kása and Csillik, 1968; Sjöstrand, 1969). Other evidence supports the view that AChE found in the axon may be synthesized locally (Clouet and Waelsch, 1961; Koenig and Koelle, 1961; Koenig, 1965; Tennyson et al., 1967; Tennyson and Brzin, 1968).

Developmental changes of AChE activity were determined by a quantitative method on isolated chick spinal ganglia (Giacobini et al., 1970): this enzymatic activity increases from the 6th to the 12th day of incubation, then it decreases steadily reaching a minimum at hatching time; in the first two days after hatching AChE activity shows once again a weak increase.

The relationship between appearance of AChE activity and beginning of the functional activity is a relevant point which can be discussed on the basis of the physiological and histochemical data now available.

In all Vertebrates sensory activity begins later than motor and association activities (Hamburger, 1964): this delay is very pronounced in the chick embryo. The first motor fibers establish provisional contacts with the anterior trunk muscles at $3^1/_2$ days of incubation (Visintini and Levi-Montalcini, 1939), and at 4 days the first spontaneous movements can be observed (Preyer, 1885; Visintini and Levi-Montalcini, 1939; Hamburger and Balaban, 1963). The peripheral processes of the spinal ganglion neuroblasts reach the skin at 6 days (Visintini and Levi-Montalcini, 1939); the first spinal collaterals of the central processes of the same cells reach the mantle layer of the alar plate at the end of the 6th day (Windle and Orr, 1934) establishing synaptic connections with association neuroblasts. A reflex circuit involving at least 3 neuroblasts (sensory, association and motor cells) is thus established, and at $6^1/_2$ to 7 days the first reflex responses can be elicited by exteroceptive stimuli (Orr and Windle, 1934; Visintini and Levi-Montalcini, 1939; Hamburger and Balaban, 1963). The first spinal collaterals of the central processes of the spinal ganglion neuroblasts reach the motor neuroblasts of the basal plate at 9 days (Visintini and Levi-Montalcini, 1939). A reflex circuit involving 2 neuroblasts (sensory and motor cells) is thus closed, and at 10 days the first localized reflex responses can be elicited by proprioceptive stimuli (Visintini and Levi-Montalcini, 1939).

From the data mentioned above it appears that in the chick embryo the synaptic function of the spinal ganglion neuroblasts does not begin before 6 days. Instead, AChE activity is detectable at 3 days.Therefore, in these neuroblasts the appearance of AChE activity is not dependent on the onset of the synaptic function. This conclusion agrees with the findings obtained by Filogamo (1960) and Taxi (1965) in other districts of the chick embryo nervous system, and with Sawyer's demonstration (1943) of a small amount of ChE in the nervous system of Amblystoma embryos before onset of motility.

The role of AChE activity in the neuroblasts and nerve cells of the spinal ganglia, generally regarded as non-cholinergic in nature (Eccles, 1948; Bremer, 1953; Feldberg, 1954), remains still unclear. A number of hypotheses regarding this matter have been put forward. It was suggested by Koelle (1955) and Feldberg

(1957) that AChE activity of the non-cholinergic nerve cells could have a "vestigial" significance. According to Nachmansohn (1959, 1961), instead, the ACh system (ChAc, ACh and AChE) would control the changes in permeability of excitable membranes in the conducting cells. Finally, the ACh system would be involved in the release of the final transmitter substance, whether it is ACh or not (Burn and Rand, 1959, 1965; Koelle, 1963; Eränkö, 1967).

Whatever the true significance of AChE activity in the spinal ganglion nerve cells, neuroblasts and neurons are the only cells in the spinal ganglion which display AChE activity; appearance of this activity in some of the ganglionic cells may, therefore, be taken as an indication of the enzymatic differentiation of these cells. The appearance of AChE activity could thus be viewed as one of the main changes which characterize the biochemical differentiation of the neuron, in parallel to the changes related to the morphological differentiation (cf. sections A and B of this chapter). The presence of AChE activity in some mitotic cells of the ganglion will be commented further on (see p. 50).

Information on the developmental changes of enzymatic activities other than that of AChE and of other chemical compounds in spinal ganglia is scanty. Developmental changes of choline acetyltransferase and monoamine oxidase activities were determined by quantitative methods on isolated chick spinal ganglia. Choline acetyltransferase activity reaches the first peak at 6 days of incubation, then it decreases. From the 12th day of incubation, this enzymatic activity increases again and reaches a second peak at 16 days, to slowly decrease thereafter (Marchisio and Consolo, 1968). Monoamine oxidase activity, after an increase from the 8th to the 12th day of incubation, does not show significant changes later on (Giacobini et al., 1970). Changes in the distribution of a nuclear histone were described in nerve cells of rat spinal ganglia during maturation (Kornguth and Tomasi, 1968). In 20-day fetuses histone appeared localized mainly in the nucleoli and also diffused in the perinuclear region; subsequently, histone could be also demonstrated in other areas of the nucleus and at the level of the Nissl substance.

F. Intercellular Relationship

Up to now we have considered the spinal ganglion neuroblasts as isolated units. However, it seems convenient to take into consideration also the mutual relationship between these cells as, in the light of present knowledge, this relationship could be of some significance in differentiation.

Above all, as Weston (1963) has pointed out, the aggregation of migrating crest cells to form the rudiment of a spinal ganglion presupposes the development of some specific affinity between the cells, since proliferation alone is not sufficient to explain the formation of a condensed structure.

At an early developmental stage, the spinal ganglion exhibits an epithelial-like structure. It is built of closely packed cells: undifferentiated cells, transitional elements between undifferentiated cells and primitive neuroblasts, and primitive neuroblasts. In particular, the ganglion lacks blood vessels and connective tissue. At this stage, two types of junction have been observed (Pannese, 1968b).

a) Adhesion Plaques. Junctions of this type (Fig. 15b) are most frequent. Along the junction the plasma membranes of the adjacent cells pursue a parallel, usually straight, course. The intercellular cleft, from 100–130 Å across, is occupied by an apparently amorphous material of moderate density. A dense, finely granular or amorphous material is condensed in the cytoplasmic matrix adjacent to the junctional area.

Junctions of this type have been observed (a) between two adjacent perikarya (Fig. 15 b), (b) between a perikaryon and an adjacent cell process, and (c) between two adjacent cell processes.

From the observations carried out on serial sections, it appears that these junctions may either occur individually or in a series. Sometimes the junction is apparent in one section only of a whole series, more frequently it can be traced through a few adjacent sections: therefore, the junctions of the first type are small, button-like structures.

Overton (1962) offered a tentative description of the sequence of events in desmosome development, as observed in the chick blastoderm: she defined three stages in such a process. The adhesion plaques described here recall the structures that Overton (1962) described in the early stage of desmosome formation. Since in the developing spinal ganglia further maturative stages of these junctions have not been observed and on the contrary they gradually disappear in further stages (see p. 47 and 48), the adhesion plaques described here seem to be junctional structures of a rather primitive kind.

b) Gap Junctions. These junctions (Fig. 15a) were previously described in the embryonic spinal ganglia as *fasciae occludentes* (Pannese, 1968b). In the sections usually employed in electron microscopy they appear less numerous than the adhesion plaques; however, since some gap junctions might escape observation because of the section thickness, it cannot be excluded that they may actually be more numerous than it appears. Gap junctions are more extensive than adhesion plaques; in section they are 0.1 to 0.2 μ in length. In serial sections it can be seen that they never encircle the whole cell body.

The over-all width of these junctions, that is, the distance between the cytoplasmic surfaces of the adjacent membranes, averages 150 Å. The intercellular cleft is about 30 Å wide. A dense, finely granular or amorphous material is condensed in the cytoplasmic matrix adjacent to the junctional area. Up to now gap junctions have only been found between adjacent perikarya (Fig. 15a), not between two adjacent cell processes or between a perikaryon and an adjacent cell process.

Adhesion plaques and gap junctions can sometimes be found arranged in junctional complexes (Fig. 15a). In section these complexes appear 1 μ or more in length but, as it can be seen in serial sections, they never encircle the whole cell. As it is the case with the gap junctions, up to now also these junctional complexes have only been observed between adjacent perikarya, and not related to cell processes.

All the types of junctions described above have been found also between mitotic cells and adjacent resting cells (Fig. 5).

As regards the functional role of the junctions, both the adhesion plaques and the gap junctions are very likely involved in cellular adhesion. This assumption is in good agreement with the data of the literature for morphologically similar junctions and with the results of experiments using hypertonic fixation.

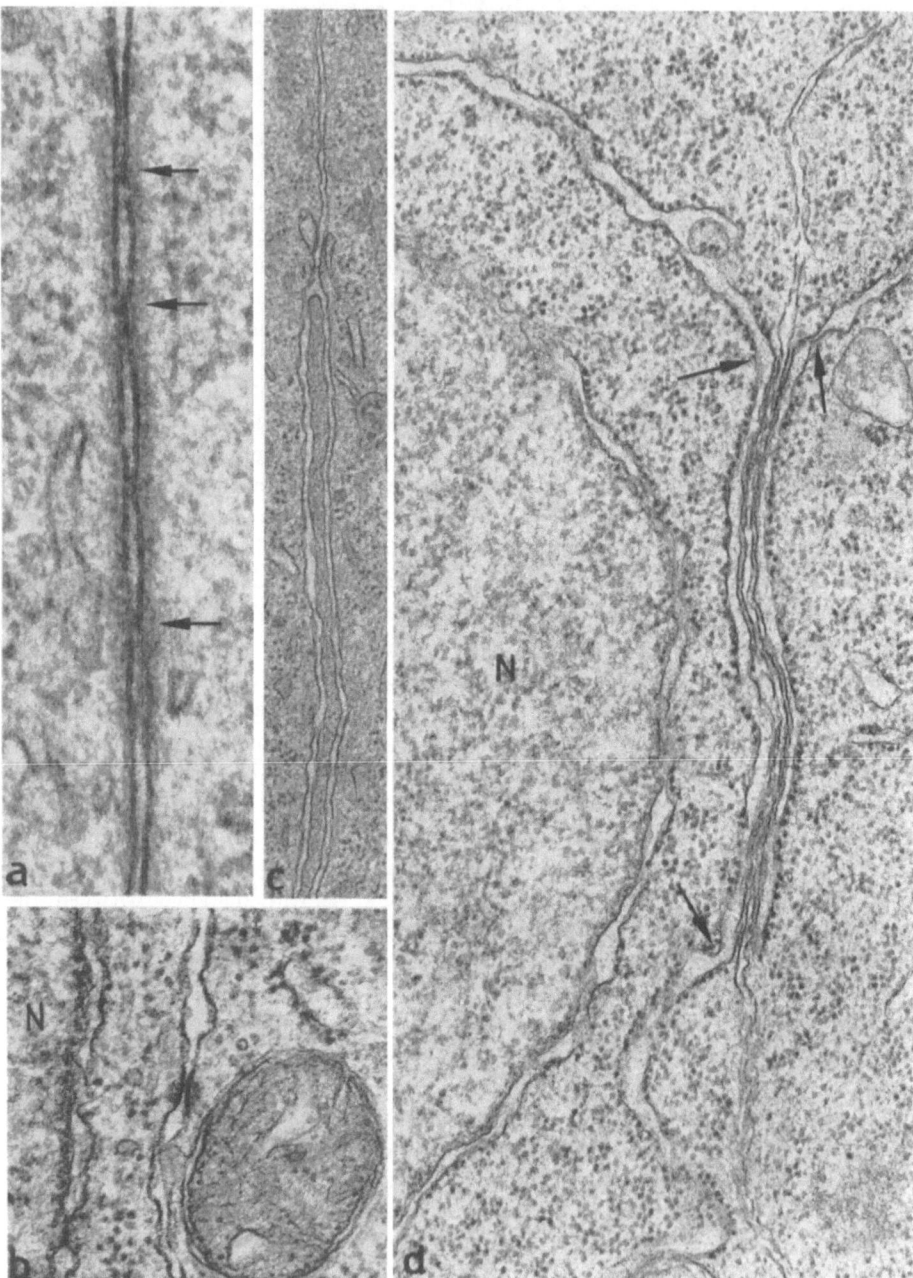

Fig. 15 a–d. Relationships between neuroblasts. Fig. a (spinal ganglion of a chick embryo: 120000 ×) shows adhesion plaques and gap junctions arranged in a junctional complex between the perikarya of two neuroblasts. Arrows point to the gap junctions in the complex. Fig. b (spinal ganglion of a chick embryo: 60000 ×) shows an adhesion plaque between a primitive neuroblast (right cell) and a transitional element between undifferentiated cell and primitive neuroblast (left cell). Both cells contain microtubules in their perikarya. N nucleus of the transitional element. Fig. c (spinal ganglion of a chick embryo: 32000 ×) shows the perikarya

In fact, under hypertonic conditions the intercellular space appears widely distended, but the cells retain their intercellular contacts at the level of the adhesion plaques and of the gap junctions. It must be emphasized that at an early developmental stage the ganglion lacks connective tissue; at this stage these junctions could play a significant role in maintaining the cell organization in the ganglion.

It is known that the gap junctions, as well as other varieties of junctions, allow ions and small molecules to pass from one cell to another (Revel and Karnovsky, 1967; Brightman and Reese, 1969; Bennett and Trinkaus, 1970). Also in the embryonic spinal ganglia the gap junctions could represent sites of exchange of ions and, possibly, of small molecules between developing cells. Such a passage of substances from one cell to the adjacent ones might have a particular role during development: according to the view advanced by Potter et al. (1966), the substances spreading directly from one cell to the adjacent ones could be of importance in the production of different effects: (a) an equivalent differentiation of all the cells of the group, if the intercellular communications are not selective, or (b) an establishment of differences between the cells, if the intercellular communications are very selective.

It should be stressed, anyhow, that the junctions observed between adjacent neuroblasts in early ganglionic development are temporary structures (Pannese, 1968b): in fact they are no longer present in later developmental stages.

These junctions disappear when development of the satellite cells commences; the expansions of the latter cells intervene between adjacent, previously closely arranged neuroblasts (Fig. 15c) thus separating them (Pannese, 1969). Junctions between neuroblasts can no longer be observed in the ganglion when each neuroblast is completely enveloped by a satellite cell sheath thereby being entirely isolated from neighboring neuroblasts.

Temporary junctions have been seldom described: e.g., in the developing tooth (Pannese, 1962), in the developing renal glomerulus (Aoki, 1967), and between mesoblastic cells and epiblast or hypoblast respectively (Hay, 1968).

At present, no hypotheses can be advanced on the disappearance mechanism of the junctions during ganglionic development; the mechanism that controls cell adhesion and, in particular, the integrity of the junctional structures has not yet been explained. It is long been known that calcium ions play a significant role in cell adhesiveness (Herbst, 1900; Meyer, 1910; Gray, 1926; Robertson, 1941; Peachey, 1964) and in maintaining the integrity of cell junctions (Sedar and Forte, 1964; Hays et al., 1965; Cassidy and Tidball, 1967; Muir, 1967); however, the mechanism of their action is still open to speculation. While Overton (1962) found half desmosomes in cells of the chick blastoderm dissociated by

of two neuroblasts which in the upper part of the figure are in mutual contact, but in the lower part are separated by the intervening cytoplasmic expansion of a satellite cell. Fig. d (spinal ganglion of a chick embryo: 45000 ×) shows confronting subsurface cisternae in two adjacent neuroblasts. At arrows the subsurface cisternae appear continuous with cisternae of the rough-surfaced endoplasmic reticulum, which lie more deeply in the perikarya. N nucleus of a neuro-blast

means of trypsin, the junctions linking adjacent neuroblasts in early ganglionic development seem to disappear completely in later developmental stages. In particular, remnants of these junctions have not been described in the neuroblasts already separated by intervening satellite cells. Therefore, the disappearance of these junctions might not depend merely on dissociation of the neuroblasts and possibly other mechanisms are required.

In the developing spinal ganglia, the junctions between the neuroblasts disappear when satellite cells develop. Information available is not yet sufficient to decide which role, if any, is played by the satellite cells in the disappearance of the junctions. If the satellite cells play an active role in the process under discussion, the data available do not evidence whether satellite cells display a mechanical or rather a chemical activity, i.e. whether or not these cells release substances which may weaken the adhesiveness of neuroblasts. Perhaps, however, the activity of the satellite cells in the disappearance of the junctions is not essential; in the material investigated by Aoki (1967), e.g., the junctions disappear independently of intervening cells. We do not even know whether the junctions described here offer some resistance to the penetration of the satellite cells. Anyhow, the resistance could not be as strong as to prevent the satellite cells from penetrating between adjacent neuroblasts and enveloping the latter completely.

G. Differentiation of the Nerve Cells, Increase in the Neuronal Population of the Spinal Ganglion, and Relationship between Mitosis and Neuronal Differentiation

a) Neuronal Differentiation. The differentiation of the neurons of the spinal ganglia is characterized by biochemical and morphological events. Biochemical changes, which up to now have not been analyzed extensively, usually precede morphological changes; the appearance of AChE activity is the best known of these biochemical events. The morphological events (summarized in Figs. 3, 16) have been more closely scrutinized. They consist of changes in cell shape, emission of two processes from the opposite poles of the cell, and marked modifications in the perikaryal structure, i.e. development of an elaborated endoplasmic reticulum with attached polysomes, enlargement of the Golgi complex, large quantitative increase in the chondriome, and appearance of numerous filaments arranged in bundles.

The major structural changes in the perikaryon of developing nerve cells of the spinal ganglia are very similar to those observed in other differentiating neurons (see, e.g., Fujita and Fujita, 1963; Lyser, 1964, 1968a; Caley and Maxwell, 1968; Meller et al., 1968; Billings, 1972). Possibly, a variety of nerve cells follow a common developmental pattern.

Some of the structural changes occurring in the perikaryon take place also in the differentiation of non-nervous cells. In fact, an elaborated rough-surfaced endoplasmic reticulum develops during the differentiation of, e.g., pancreatic acinar cells (Munger, 1958), cnidoblasts of Hydra (Slautterback and Fawcett, 1959), and gland cells of Hydra (Lentz, 1965), and bundles of filaments morphologically similar to the neurofilaments become evident during neuroglial cell

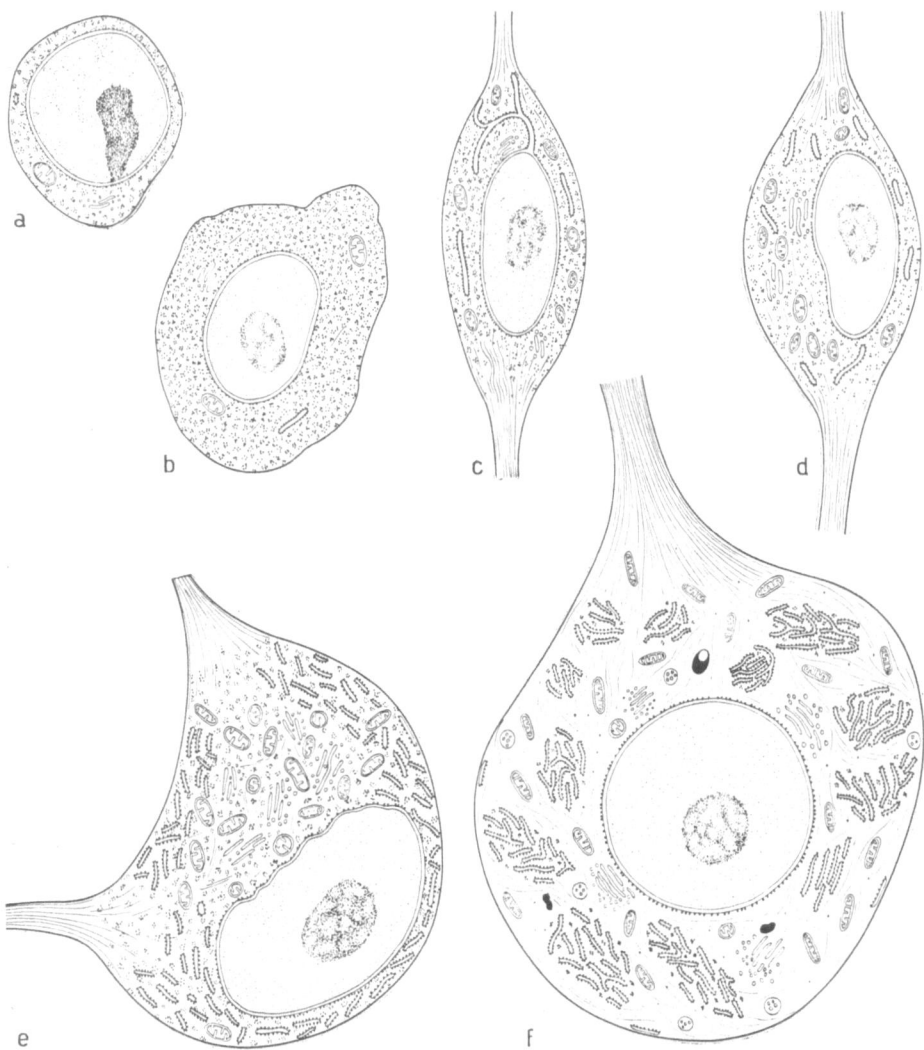

Fig. 16a–f. Diagram showing some major events occurring at the electron microscope level during the differentiation and maturation of a spinal ganglion nerve cell. a, undifferentiated cell; b, transitional element between undifferentiated cell and primitive neuroblast; c, primitive neuroblast; d, transitional element between the primitive and the intermediate neuroblast; e, intermediate neuroblast; d, pseudo-unipolar nerve cell

differentiation (Lyser, 1971). Therefore, none of the events listed above is sufficient by itself to characterize neuronal differentiation, although they might altogether characterize this process.

The nuclear envelope seems to participate to more than one of the morphological events which take place in the differentiation of ganglionic neurons. In fact (see p. 34, 35, and 37 to 39), the nuclear envelope seems to be involved in the biosynthesis of membrane for the rough-surfaced endoplasmic reticulum, as well as for the Golgi complex and mitochondria. Formation of an elaborated endo-plasmic reticulum, enlargement of the Golgi complex, and increase in the chon-driome are some of the morphological events which characterize neuroblastic differentiation at the electron microscope level; it seems therefore warranted to conclude that nuclear envelope plays an important role in sensory neuron differentiation.

It is well known that the formation of membrane may be considered to be a major function of the nuclear envelope (Kessel, 1971). In the spinal ganglion neuroblasts at an early developmental stage the nuclear envelope seems capable of producing simultaneously membranes having the capacity to differentiate into organelles with different structural and functional characteristics. Something similar has also been described in other cell classes (see, e.g., Kessel, 1971).

Conceivably, the nuclear envelope contains informations to regulate and con-trol its activity of membrane production. Different zones of the same nuclear envelope must evidently contain different informations. Factors controlling and directing the activity of the different areas of the nuclear envelope are as yet unknown and they may be hypothesized only: it may be postulated, e.g., that information coming from the nucleus reaches the nuclear envelope, thus controlling and directing its membrane forming activity. In this connection, the nuclear envelope appears well situated to ensure the early incorporation of information (Locke, 1964) coming from the genes and relevant to the structural and functional fate of the membranes.

b) Increase in the Neuronal Population and Relationship between Mitosis and Neuronal Differentiation. The increase in the neuronal population takes place through the following two processes:

α) differentiation of undifferentiated cells, which, on their part, are capable of mitotic division (see Chapter II);

β) multiplication of transitional elements between the undifferentiated cell and the primitive neuroblast (Fig. 5), i.e., multiplication of cells which already undergo morphological differentiation toward the neuron.

The event listed under β together with the fact that mitotic cells can display AChE activity (see p. 41–42) throw a new light on the relationship between mitosis and neuronal differentiation. It was originally maintained that neuroblastic diffe-rentiation of the daughter cells could only begin after the end of the parent cell division. Therefore, mitotic cells in the nervous tissue were formerly regarded as fully undifferentiated elements. This can no longer be maintained as transitional elements between the undifferentiated cell and the primitive neuroblast (i.e. cells which have already commenced their morphological differentiation) can be found in mitosis (not only in spinal ganglia, but also in the retina of the chick embryo: Sechrist, 1969) and also cells displaying AChE activity (i.e. cells which have already commenced their biochemical differentiation) can be found in mitosis (Pannese *et al.*, 1971).

The occurrence of mitotic cells which synthesize AChE is another case that should be added to the examples already known of dividing cells which syn-thesize specialized proteins. Here are some: actively dividing blasts (i.e. plasma cells precursors) can synthesize antibodies (De Petris and Karlsbad, 1965); cultured fibroblasts synthesize collagen very rapidly in exponentially growing cultures (Priest and Davies, 1969; Manner, 1971); both smooth and cardiac muscle cells undergo mitosis while contractile proteins are synthesized (smooth muscle cells: Bennett and Cobb, 1969; Cobb and Bennett, 1970; cardiac muscle cells: DeHaan, 1967; Manasek, 1968; Rumyantsev and Snigirevskaya, 1968; Weinstein and Hay, 1970; Oberpriller and Oberpriller, 1971; Przybylski, 1971; Hay and Low, 1972); primitive erythroblasts in the circulating blood continue to divide while synthesizing hemoglobin (Campbell *et al.*, 1971). These and other similar findings question the long held view that cell proliferation and synthesis of specialized proteins are mutually exclusive activities.

V. Degenerative Events in Developing Ganglia

Collin (1906) first reported the occurrence of degenerating cells in the ventral horn of the chick embryo spinal cord. Cellular degeneration was then observed repeatedly also in other sites of the developing nervous system including the spinal ganglia, and some authors pointed out the role of this phenomenon in morphogenesis (see Glücksmann, 1951 and Saunders, 1966 for a review). A brief list of the authors who studied with the light microscope degenerative events in developing spinal ganglia and the zoological species used are reported in Table 1.

Schedule and localization of this phenomenon in the chick embryo were illustrated in detail by Hamburger and Levi-Montalcini (1949). The degenerating cells are numerous during the 5th and 6th incubation day, then they decrease in number and finally disappear at the end of the 7th day of incubation. The large brachial and lumbosacral ganglia which innervate wing and leg buds are either free of degeneration, or they show a limited number of degenerating cells; the latter are numerous in the cervical and thoracic ganglia. The degenerating cells are localized in the lateroventral region of the ganglion, that is occupied

Table 1

Author (or authors)	Year	Zoological species
Collin	1906	chick embryo
Nicolas	unpublished observations reported by Collin (1906)	rabbit embryo
Hett	1925	man embryo
Ernst	1926	chick, duck, mole, rabbit, mouse, and man embryos
Glücksmann	1934	Birds and Mammals
Hamburger and Levi-Montalcini	1949	chick embryo
Hughes	1955	chick embryo
Stefanelli	1955	chick embryo
Palladini	1961	Japanese quail embryo
Prestige	1965	Xenopus tadpoles

by the early differentiating large neuroblasts; therefore, the authors maintain that the degeneration affects these cells only. Wing or leg bud extirpation results in degenerative cellular changes also in the large brachial and lumbo-sacral ganglia which are normally spared from this phenomenon.

In the spinal ganglia of the Japanese quail a massive cell degeneration occurs between the 6th and the 12th day of incubation (Palladini, 1961). The degenerating cells are localized predominantly in the lateroventral region of the ganglion. During the early stages of the process the affected cell appears deeply baso-philic, then one or two Feulgen-positive granules are observed in the area pre-viously occupied by the nucleus and toward the end of the process the whole cell appears as a spherical mass which stains deeply with iron hematoxylin.

In the spinal ganglia of Xenopus tadpoles the cell degeneration rate is extremely high from stage 53 to 59, i.e. for a period of over 3 weeks (Prestige, 1965). The degeneration of a spinal ganglion neuroblast takes about 3 hours and two-thirds of the nerve cells degenerate during differentiation.

The light microscopy studies mentioned have thus clearly established that also in the spinal ganglia, as in other districts of the nervous system, many nerve cells are formed that do not survive. Cell degeneration, which is probably influenced by the peripheral field of innervation, could be one of the factors that regulate the size of the cell population of the ganglion (Hamburger and Levi-Montalcini, 1949; Glücksmann, 1951).

Some ultrastructural aspects of degenerating neuroblasts of embryonic spinal ganglia have recently been described (Tennyson, 1970b; Birks and Weldon, 1971; Weis, 1971), but, as far as I know, a systematic study of this degenerative process at the electron microscope level is still lacking.

In chick embryo spinal ganglia most images of degenerating neuroblasts can be classified in terms of stages of degeneration, so that the following sequence of events can be tentatively reconstructed. In an early stage the cells undergoing degeneration show an increase in density of both the nucleoplasm and cytoplasmic matrix (Fig. 17a); the nuclear envelope is intact and the nucleolus is still recogniz-able and exhibits the usual structure. Also subsequent changes involve both the nucleus and the cytoplasm. One or more dense, spherical inclusions appear in the nucleus (Fig. 17a) of many affected cells. These inclusions have a maximum dia-meter of 2.5 μ in section, show a finely granular texture, and sharp boundaries, although they lack a limiting membrane; a nucleolus, with a modified structure, can sometimes be distinguished near these inclusions. As it will be recalled further on, these inclusions can still be observed in very advanced stages of degene-ration. Dense particles appear in the nucleus. An extensive vacuolation is evident

Fig. 17a–c. Cells at an early stage of degeneration (spinal ganglion of a chick embryo). Fig. a (16000 ×) shows a degenerating cell which exhibits an increased density of both the nucleoplasm and cytoplasmic matrix. The nuclear envelope is intact and a dense inclusion (i) is evident inside the nucleus (N). Several vacuoles with a clear content, clusters of mitochondria (m) some of which appear altered, and ribosomal crystals (arrows) are recognizable in the cytoplasm. The degenerating cell is surrounded by elements showing a normal structure. nu, nucleus of a surrounding cell. Fig. b (33000 ×) shows a part of a degenerating cell in which two bundles of closely packed filaments, and both normal and altered (arrows) mitochondria can be seen. Fig. c (50000 ×) shows a part of a degenerating cell in which a large amount of ribo-somes can be seen. nu, nucleus of a surrounding cell

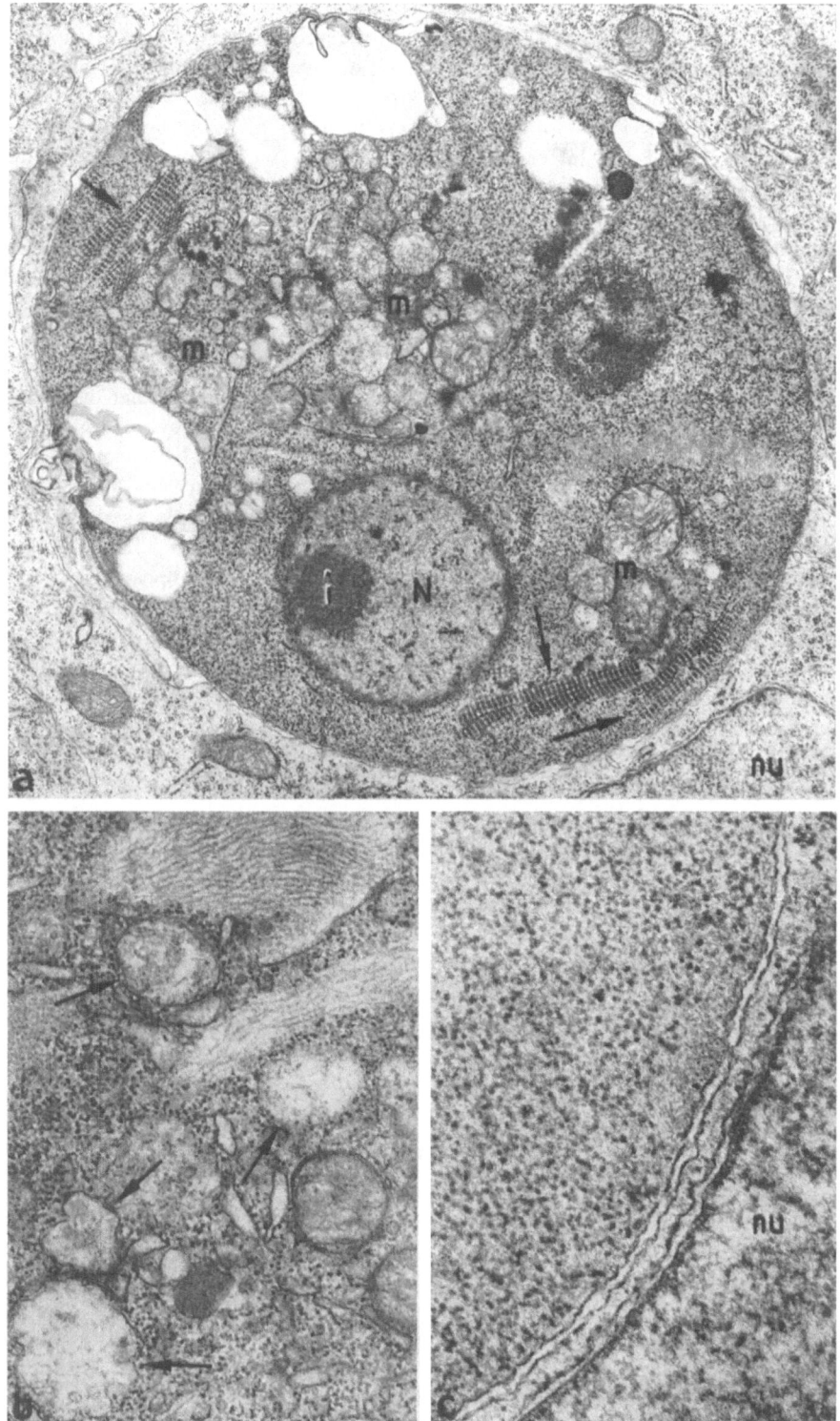

Fig. 17 a–c

in the cytoplasm (Fig. 17a); the vacuoles are bounded by a single membrane, exhibit a clear content, and their maximum diameter in section is less than 1 μ. Some of these vacuoles seem to open at the cell surface; perhaps material which was previously contained inside the cell is extruded by means of these vacuoles. The Golgi complex is no longer recognizable, while mitochondria can still be identified: some of the latter may appear normal, while others are evidently altered (Fig. 17a, b). Altered mitochondria can display focal to extensive dissolution of the outer membrane thus appearing limited more or less extensively by a single membrane, as it was also observed in an axonal dystrophy produced by Vitamin E deficiency (Schochet, 1971). Other mitochondrial alterations affect both cristae and matrix: the cristae can appear reduced in number and show various degrees of disorganization, while the matrix may show a decreased density. Discrete bundles of closely packed filaments are evident (Fig. 17b). The cytoplasmic area occupied by these bundles of filaments is devoid of other organelles, and so it stands out sharply being lighter than the remaining cytoplasm. Large amounts of ribosomes are found in these cells (Fig. 17c). Although polysomes can be distinguished here and there, most of the free[2] ribosomes are usually so tightly packed that it is difficult to establish whether they are arranged as single units (monosomes) or they are still in the usual polysomic configuration. The membrane-attached ribosomes may retain the usual arrangement, or appear as rows of granules regularly spaced along the profiles of the endoplasmic reticulum membranes.

In a further stage the nuclear envelope appears fragmented; the remnants of the nuclear envelope are sometimes arranged in pairs, as they can also be seen in mitotic cells. The nuclear and cytoplasmic structures do not yet appear intermingled. In this stage the vacuoles with a clear content seem less numerous but larger than before, their maximum diameter reaching 2 μ in section. Probably each of these vacuoles arises by confluence of a few smaller vacuoles (Fig. 18a). Successively the remnants of the nuclear envelope are no longer recognizable, and the nuclear and cytoplasmic structures appear intermingled. The dense, spherical inclusions seen inside the nucleus before, become prominent in these degenerating cells.

In a still more advanced stage of the process, seemingly empty spaces appear intermingled with dense spaces (Fig. 19a). The apparently empty spaces look sometimes bounded by membrane fragments, and they might be derived from the vacuoles with a clear content which do not empty at the cell surface and whose limiting membrane undergoes fragmentation. In the dense spaces, single ribosomes and mitochondria showing various degrees of degradation are discernible (Fig. 19a). Some mitochondria show the alterations already described, others appear transformed in

Fig. 18a–c. Cells at an intermediate stage of degeneration (spinal ganglion of a chick embryo). Fig. a (21 000 ×) shows a degenerating cell lacking the nuclear envelope. A large, dense inclusion (*i*), several vacuoles with a clear content, and ribosomal crystals (arrows) are evident in this cell. Note that some of the vacuoles contain membrane fragments and that vacuoles 1 and 2 and respectively 3 and 4 seem to be confluent. The degenerating cell is surrounded by elements showing a normal structure. *nu*, nucleus of a surrounding cell. Fig. b and c (90000 ×) show two different views of ribosomal crystals at a higher magnification

2 See note on p. 10.

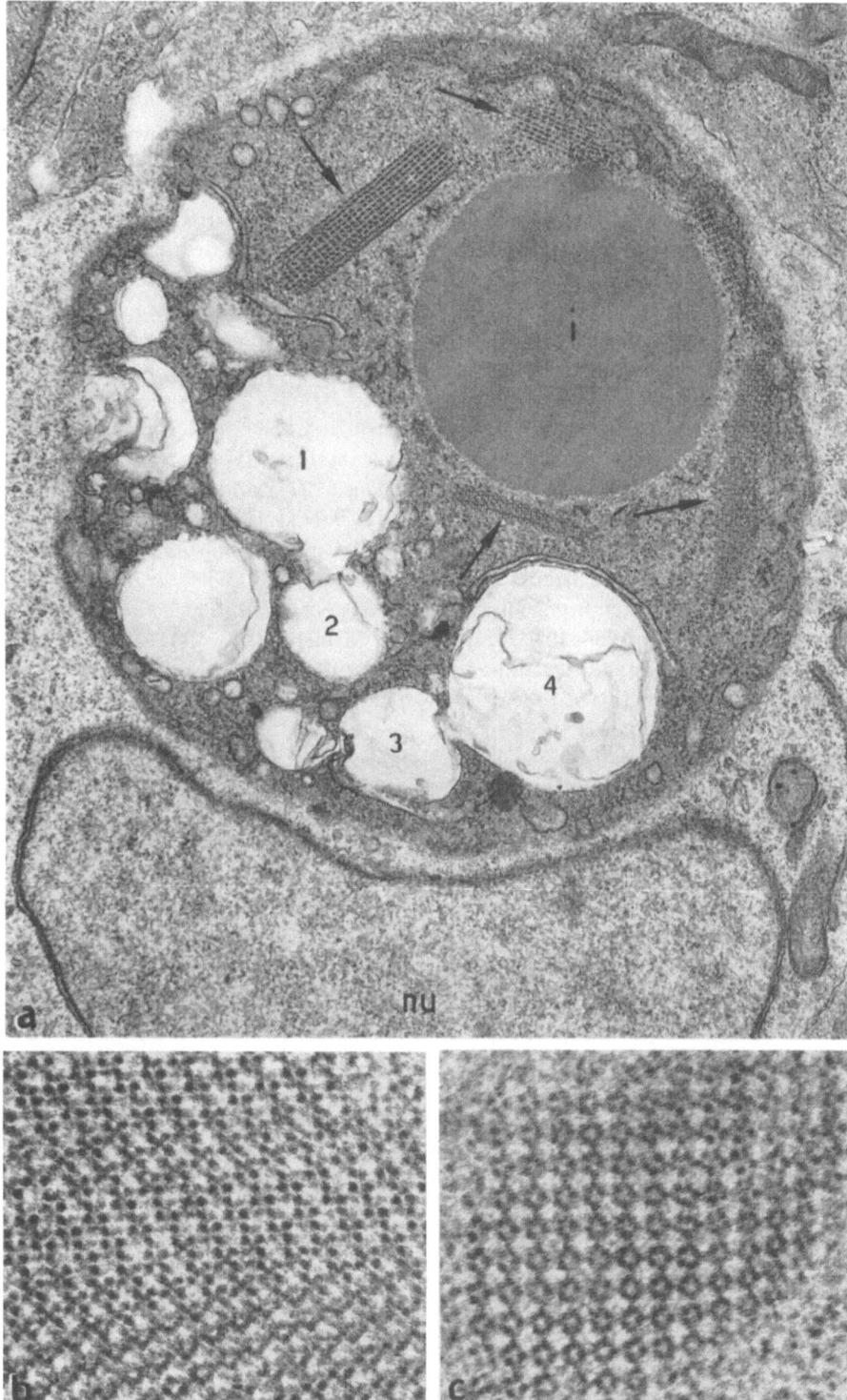

Fig. 18 a–c

spherical vesicles limited by a single membrane: they contain a scarce granular material dispersed within the clear matrix. Sometimes a row of ribosomes appears arranged over the limiting membrane of the altered mitochondrion (Fig. 19a). Gradually the apparently empty spaces extend relatively to the dense parts. The remaining mitochondria are not easily identifiable; very dense deposits are now placed over their limiting membrane instead of the ribosomes (Fig. 19c).

In the final stage of the process the degenerated cells appear rather light and contain aggregates of flocculent material and membrane fragments (Fig. 19b). Sometimes they still show the dense inclusions that in the early stage of the process could be seen inside the nucleus. These inclusions may retain the same characteristics as in the early stage of the process, or they may appear modified. In fact, they may appear more dense, irregularly shaped and smaller than before, or they seem to consist of a dense "cortex" and a lighter core.

Ribosomal crystals are evident in all the stages of the process (Figs. 17a, 18a, b, c, 19b). These crystals were already described in degenerating neuroblasts of the spinal ganglia of the chick embryo (Goldsmith et al., 1967; Weston, 1970; Birks and Weldon, 1971; Weis, 1971) and in degenerating cells of the early chick blastoderm (Bellairs, 1961). This kind of crystal was described also in neuroblasts of the chick embryo spinal ganglia cultured in vitro (Crain et al., 1964), in eggs of lizards (Ghiara et al., 1966; Taddei, 1972) as well as in various tissues of embryos submitted to hypothermic treatment (Byers, 1966, 1967; Barbieri et al., 1968, 1970; Maraldi and Barbieri, 1969). In the spinal ganglia, these ribosomal crystals seem to be very resistant to autolysis as in very advanced stages of the degenerative process they remain the only structures recognizable among the cellular debris.

To analyze the role played by lysosomes in the degeneration of the spinal ganglion neuroblasts, the electron microscope histochemical technique of Gomori for the demonstration of acid phosphatase was applied to chick embryo spinal ganglia (Pannese et al., unpublished observations). Degenerating neuroblasts at the early stages of the process still contain recognizable cell organelles (e.g. mitochondria and endoplasmic reticulum cisternae) and show reaction product sharply localized within the lysosomes. The degenerated neuroblasts at the final stage of the process are free of identifiable cell organelles and show a more diffuse pattern of the reaction product. These findings suggest that the early degenerative changes in the spinal ganglion neuroblasts may not be related to a lysosomal activity while

Fig. 19a–c. Cells at very advanced stages of degeneration (spinal ganglion of a chick embryo). Fig. a (20000 ×) shows a degenerating cell in which dense spaces appear intermingled with seemingly empty spaces containing membrane fragments. A dense inclusion (i) and some altered mitochondria (m) are recognizable in this cell. A row of ribosomes (arrowed) can be seen arranged over the limiting membrane of some of the altered mitochondria. nu nucleus of a surrounding cell. Fig. b (20000 ×) shows a degenerating cell at the final stage of the process. This cell, which appears rather light, contains a dense inclusion (i), a ribosomal crystal (arrow), aggregates of flocculent material, and membrane fragments. The degenerating cell is surrounded by elements showing a normal structure. nu nucleus of a surrounding cell. Fig. c (24000 ×) shows some altered mitochondria (m) with dense deposits placed over their limiting membrane, in a degenerating cell at a very advanced stage of the process

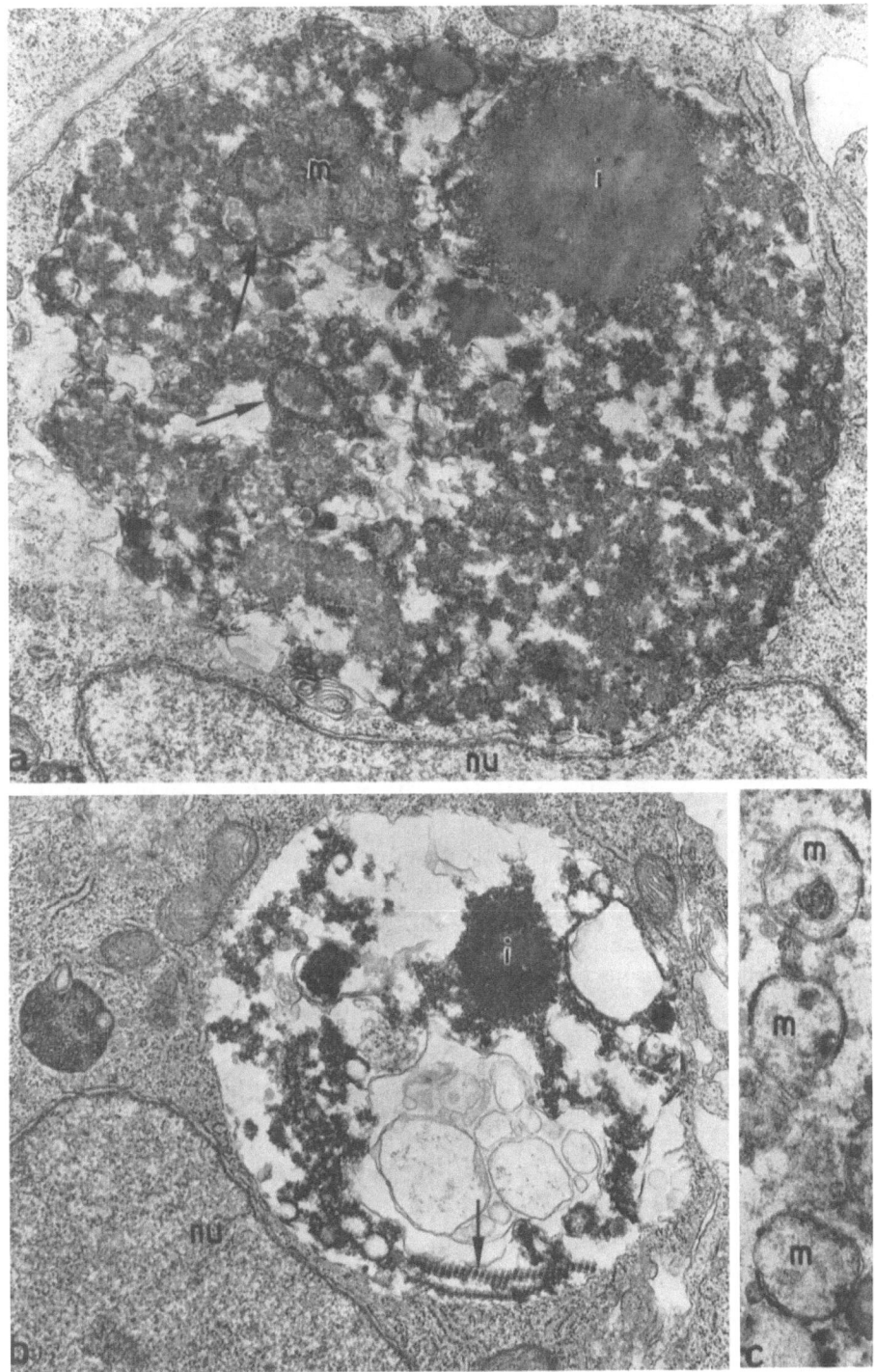

Fig. 19 a–c

the late degenerative alterations are probably dependent upon the release of hydro-lytic enzymes from lysosomes.

The type of cell, or cells involved in the removal of the remnants of degenerated neuroblasts has not yet been determined. The presence of macrophages in chick embryo spinal ganglia affected by cell degeneration was observed in light micro-scope preparations (Hamburger and Levi-Montalcini, 1949). According to Tenny-son (1970b), however, cellular debris in embryonic ganglia would be taken up by satellite cells; therefore, these cells would be capable of phagocytic activity during early development. Systematic studies on this problem are wanting.

VI. Development of Satellite Cells, Interstitial Spaces, and Blood Vessels

1. Development of Satellite Cells. Light Microscopy

Little information has been produced with the use of the light microscope on the early development of the satellite cells in spinal ganglia.

In the rabbit, Morpurgo and Tirelli (1893) found a very few star-shaped satellite cells in spinal ganglia of 9 mm embryos; they observed also dividing satellite cells up to the first weeks after birth. Levi (1908), who studied ganglionic development in many species, came to the conclusion that satellite cells appear later than neuroblasts. In chick embryo spinal ganglia Brizzee (1949) noticed satellite cells from the 7th incubation day, and observed images suggesting the formation of a perineuronal envelope from the 15th day. He found that the development of the perineuronal envelope was nearly completed in the 10-day chick. Again, in the chick embryo spinal ganglia Yates (1961) found satellite cells since the 6th incubation day and dividing cells with a low cytoplasmic RNA content (i. e. very likely dividing satellite cells) from the 9th incubation day.

As regards the development of the Schwann cells within the spinal ganglion, the myelination was found to begin *in vivo* at about the 12th day and progress rapidly during the 13th to 15th day in the chick embryo (Peterson and Murray, 1955). The myelin formation was investigated in more detail by the same authors with the light microscope in chick embryo spinal ganglia cultured *in vitro*.

2. Development of Satellite Cells. Electron Microscopy

Electron microscopical observations have confirmed that satellite cells appear after neuroblasts during spinal ganglia development. However, satellite cells can be recognized by electron microscopy earlier than by light microscopy.

The development of satellite cells in spinal ganglia has been extensively studied with the electron microscope in the chick by Pannese (1969), and in

Fig. 20. Star-shaped satellite cell (sc), whose body is located in the center of a group of neuroblasts (spinal ganglion of a chick embryo: 19000 ×). The cytoplasmic expansions of the satellite cell intervene between the neighboring neuroblasts (N_1 to N_5). In this section the neuroblasts N_1 and N_2 and respectively N_3 and N_4 are still in mutual contact. Arrow points to a pinocytotic vesicle in the neuroblast N_2

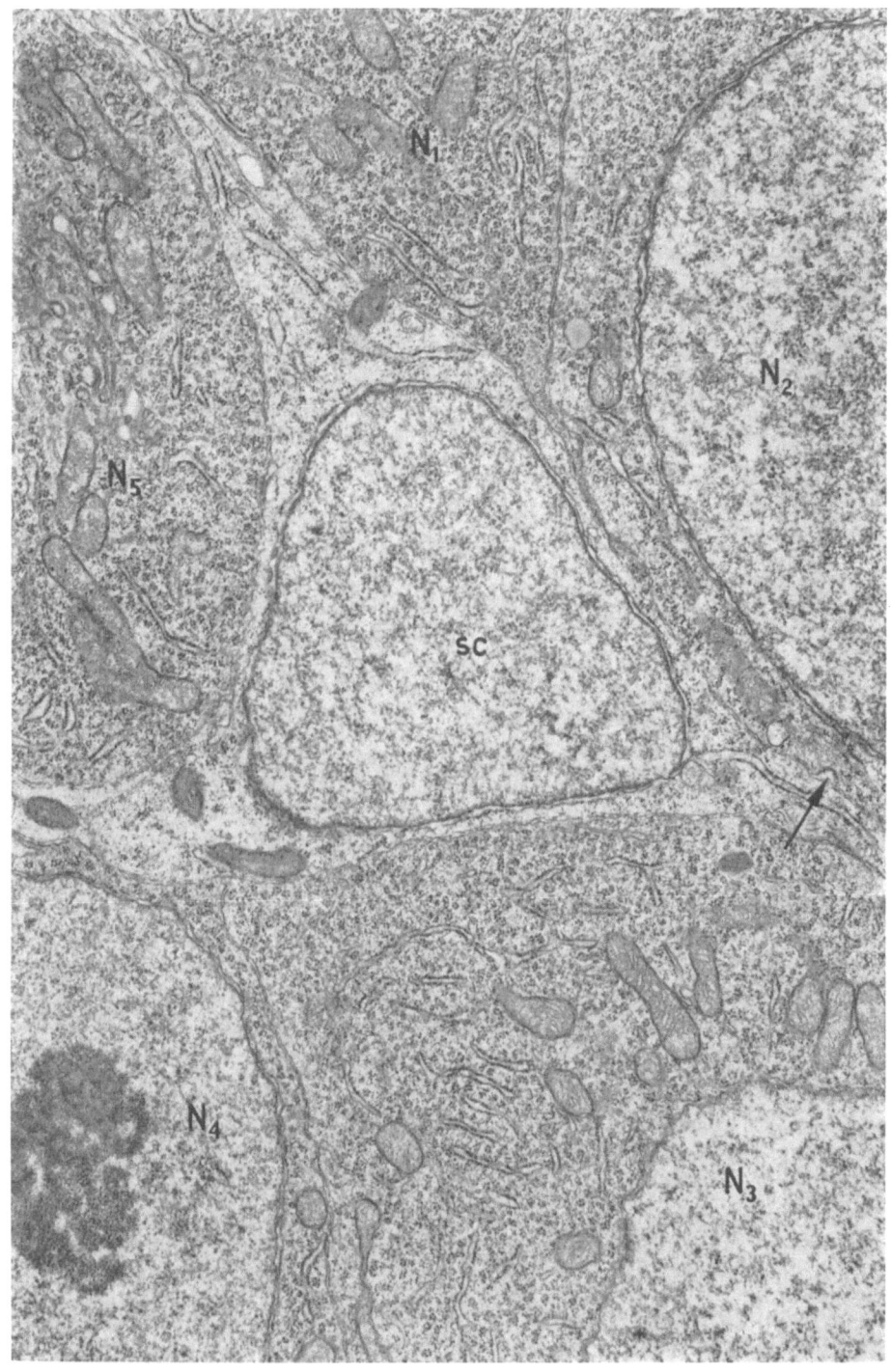

Fig. 20

the rabbit by Tennyson (1970 b). On the basis of these studies the following developmental stages can be traced.

a) When satellite cells are first detectable in the ganglion, they appear star-shaped in section, and they consist of a nucleated body with several attenuated cytoplasmic expansions (Fig. 20). The body of each satellite cell is located in the center of a group of neuroblasts and its cytoplasmic expansions radiate out intervening between neighboring neuroblasts. Thus at this stage each satellite cell is related to several neuroblasts and each of its cytoplasmic expansions contacts at least two neuroblasts (Fig. 20). At this stage the neuroblasts largely outnumber the satellite cells, so that only some of the neuroblasts come in direct contact with satellite cells, the majority of the neuroblasts remaining in mutual contact.

The satellite cell nucleus is nearly triangular or more irregularly-shaped in section. The nucleoplasm is a little more dense than its counterpart in the neuroblast; the chromatin occurs in small clumps scattered throughout the nucleoplasm and in a thin peripheral accumulation. Free ribosomal clusters, one or two short rough-surfaced profiles of the endoplasmic reticulum, a few mitochondria, Golgi complex and some microtubules (200 to 300 Å in diameter) are usually seen in every section of the satellite cell body (Fig. 20); lipid droplets, multivesicular bodies, dense bodies, and centrioles are occasionally observed.

The satellite cell expansions (300 to 2 000 Å in thickness) consist of a matrix limited by a plasma membrane (Fig. 15 c). In the matrix, free ribosomal clusters, microtubules, and an occasional filament (less than 100 Å in thickness) may be found. Pinocytotic vesicles, mostly of the coated type, are often present near the plasma membrane. The plasma membrane of the attenuated expansions of the satellite cell follows often a wrinkled course. If this aspect does not depend on an artifactual retraction of a thin expansion produced by the technical procedure and it is related instead to a dynamic condition preexisting in the living state, then the attenuated expansions of the satellite cells observed at this stage might be interpreted as ondulating membranes.

b) In the successive developmental stage satellite cells appear more numerous than in the preceding stage. At this stage only small areas of the perikaryal surface of the neuroblast are not invested by satellite cells (Figs. 6 a, 8, 9) and here and there a satellite cell sheet, consisting of two adjoining cytoplasmic expansions, may be found intervening between two adjacent neuroblasts (Fig. 6 a).

Isolated cilia lacking fibers or tubular structures in their central portion are sometimes seen in the body of the satellite cells (Fig. 9) in addition to the structures already existing in the preceding stage. Isolated cilia can be sometimes observed also in the next developmental stage and in adult specimens. The membranous expansions of the satellite cells appear now more extensive, thicker and richer in organelles; in fact, they may contain also some mitochondria, profiles of the rough-surfaced endoplasmic reticulum, and dense bodies.

Here and there, adjoining satellite cells appear mutually linked by adhering and gap junctions. Among these junctions, those linking satellite cells which in the next developmental stage will envelope different nerve cells (Fig. 24 a) are transitory (Pannese, 1969).

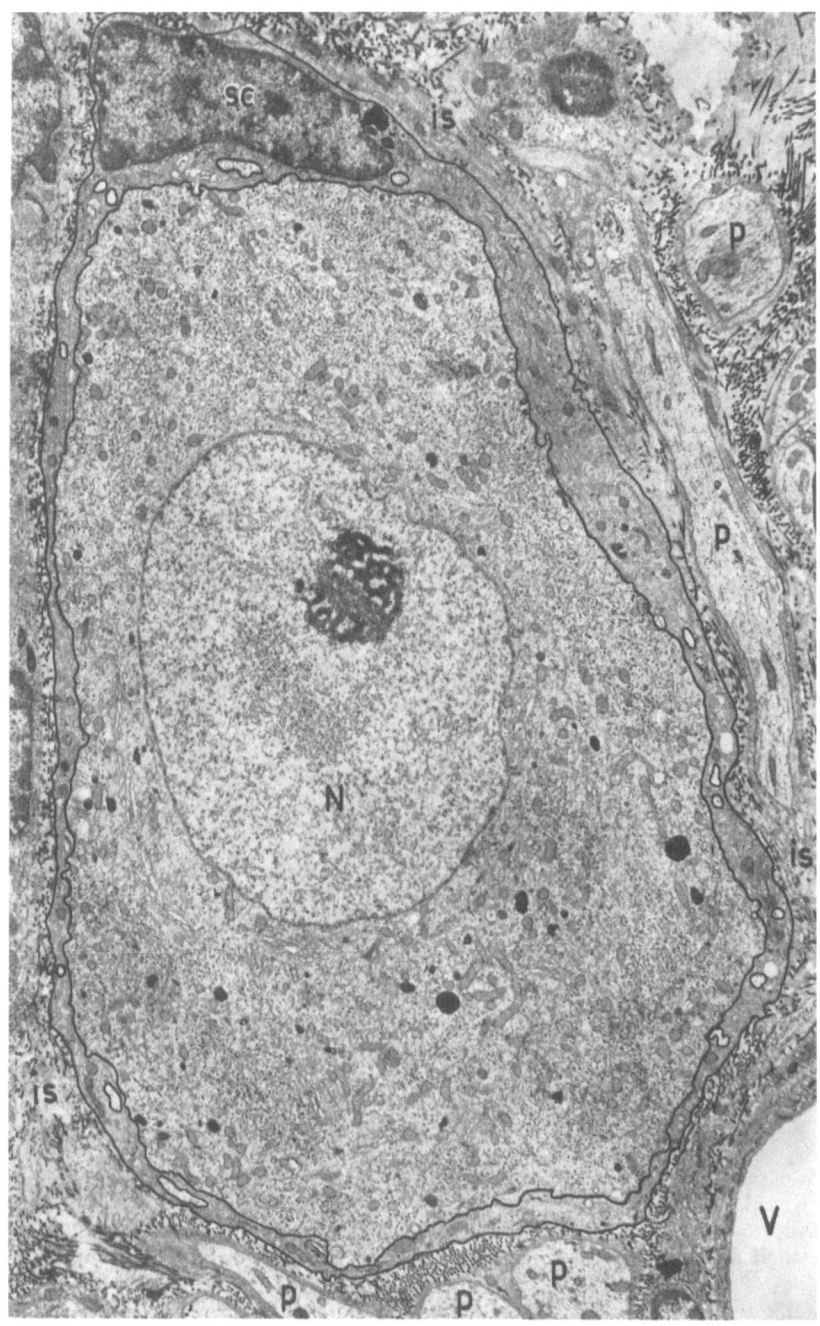

Fig. 21. Nerve cell body of a mature neuron (spinal ganglion of an adult rabbit: 7500 ×) completely enveloped by its satellite cell sheath, which is in turn completely sur-rounded by the interstitial space (*is*). The neuron-satellite cell boundary and the outer contour of the satellite cell sheath are outlined in ink to show their complicated courses. *N* nerve cell nucleus, *p* nerve cell processes, *sc* satellite cell nucleus, *V* blood vessel

c) In a later developmental stage each nerve cell is completely enveloped by a satellite cell sheath. Whereas in some regions the sheath is formed by one single cell layer, in other regions the same sheath consists of some overlapping cytoplasmic expansions. Passing from stage *a* to this stage, the satellite cell changes its earlier star shape to the mature flattened shape, probably by retracting some of its cytoplasmic expansions. While at stage *a* one satellite cell was related to several neuroblasts, in this stage one or more satellite cells appear related to one nerve cell only, so that now satellite cells outnumber nerve cells. Mitotic satellite cells are evident (Pannese, 1969). Each mitotic satellite cell belongs to a distinct perineuronal sheath and it appears in direct contact with one nerve cell only. Hence, satellite cells may undergo mitosis after differentiation, as Schwann cells of peripheral nerves (Peters and Muir, 1959; Cravioto, 1965; Diner, 1965; Asbury, 1967). The rough-surfaced endoplasmic reticulum and the Golgi complex of the satellite cell appear increased in volume in comparison to their counterparts in the preceding stages.

d) At the end of body growth, satellite cells show the same general characteristics as in the preceding stage. Between the two stages quantitative differences only can be noticed: in fact, in adult specimens (Figs. 21, 22 b, 24 c) the satellite cell sheaths are thicker and consist of a greater number of cells in comparison to the preceding stage. Also at this stage adhering and gap junctions link satellite cells of the same perineuronal sheath. These junctions increase the adhesion between the satellite cells; gap junctions could be also sites of exchange of ions and, possibly, small molecules between satellite cells of the same perineuronal sheath.

The structure of Schwann cells and that of the myelin sheaths have been investigated with the electron microscope in rat spinal ganglia cultured *in vitro* by Bunge *et al.* (1967) and they have been found similar to their counterparts in other regions of the peripheral nervous system.

Fig. 22 a–e. Neuron-satellite cell boundary. Fig. a (spinal ganglion of a chick embryo: 24 000 ×) shows the relatively smooth boundaries between the perikarya of two neuroblasts and a satellite cell in the stage in which the satellite cells are first detectable in the ganglion. A centriole (*c*), Golgi complexes (*G*), rough-surfaced profiles of the endoplasmic reticulum, and microtubules can be seen in the satellite cell body. Arrow points to a subsurface cisterna in a neuroblast. *N* nuclei of the neuroblasts, *sc* satellite cell nucleus. Fig. b (spinal ganglion of an adult rabbit: 16 000 ×) shows the complicated course of the boundary between the perikaryon (*nc*) of a mature neuron and its satellite cell sheath (*sc*). The complicated course of this boundary is mainly due to finger-like projections (*) arising from the perikaryon. The irregular boundary between the satellite cell sheath (*sc*) and the interstitial space (*is*) can also be seen in this figure. Fig. c (spinal ganglion of an adult rabbit: 24 000 ×) shows the complicated course of the boundary between the process (*p*) of a mature neuron and its satellite cell sheath (*sc*). The complicated course of this boundary is mainly due to finger-like projections (*) arising from the neuronal process. Neurofilaments, rare microtubules, glycogen granules, and profiles of the smooth-surfaced endoplasmic reticulum can be seen in the neuronal process. *is*, interstitial space. Fig. d (spinal ganglion of a chick embryo: 100 000 ×) shows a button-like, adhering junction (arrow) at the boundary between the perikaryon of a neuroblast (lower cell) and a satellite cell (upper cell). Fig. e (spinal ganglion of an adult rabbit: 100 000 ×) shows a button-like, adhering junction (arrow) at the boundary between the perikaryon of a mature neuron (lower cell) and a satellite cell (upper cell)

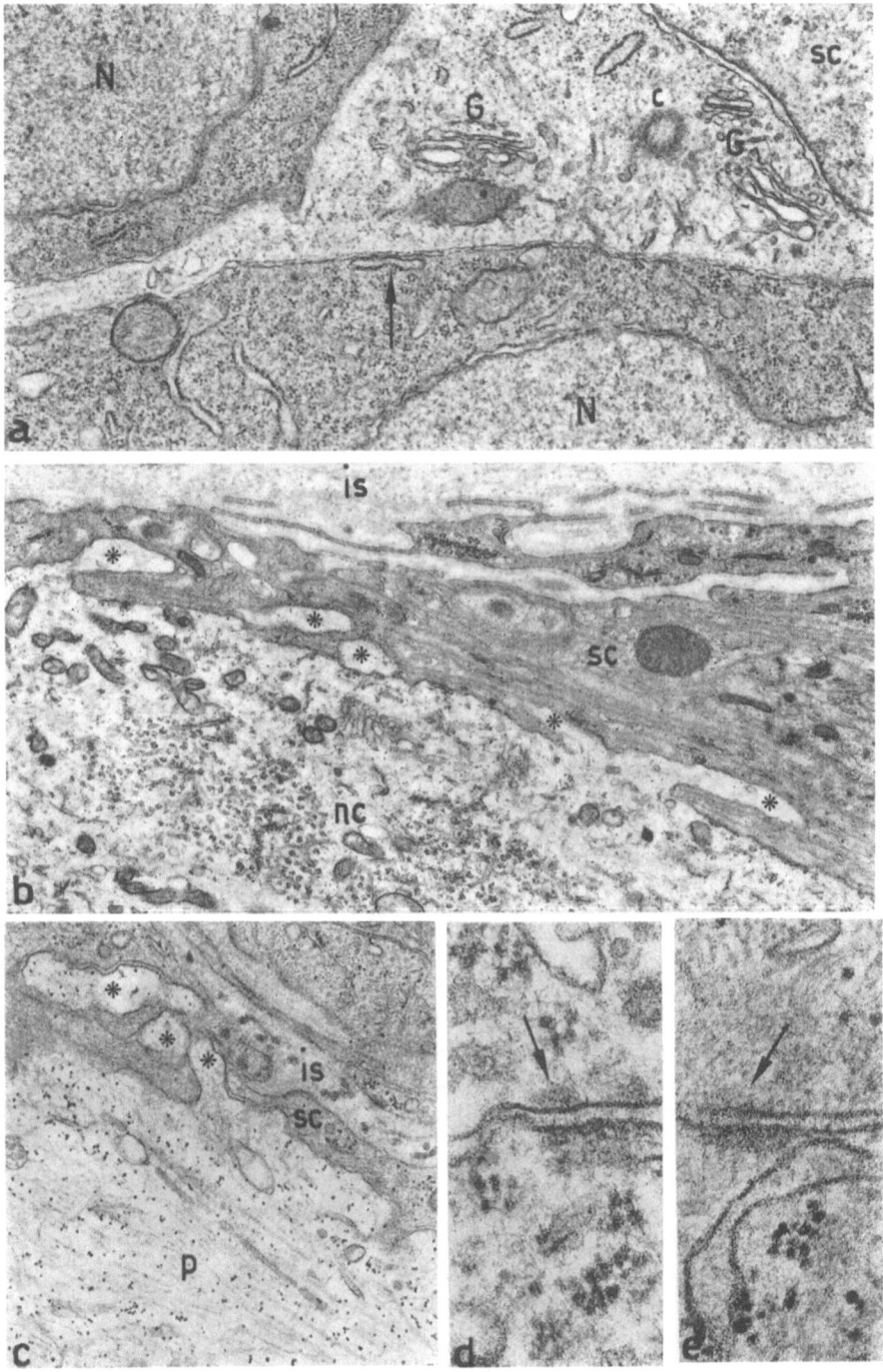

Fig. 22

3. Neuron-Satellite Cell Boundary

When satellite cells are first detectable in the ganglion (stage a), the outline of the neuronal perikaryon appears relatively smooth (Figs. 20, 22a), but already in the following stage (stage b) this contour may sometimes show a complicated course, due to finger-like projections arising from the perikaryon. These projections invaginate the apposed contour of the satellite cell or extend along the cleft between neuroblast and satellite cell. Projections arising from the satellite cell may also be observed, although less frequently.

In the successive developmental stages the perikaryal projections become more and more numerous (Figs. 21, 22b); moreover, the perikaryal plasma membrane shows also deep infoldings, which were not detectable earlier. Thus, during development the perikaryal boundary becomes gradually more irregular and complicated (Pannese, 1969; Yamadori, 1970); thereby, the surface area of the perikaryon increases much more than it would through the mere increase in volume of the nerve cell body. As a great deal of neuronal exchanges occur at the perikaryal surface, the marked increase in area of this surface is probably instrumental for the metabolism of the ganglionic nerve cell.

Pinocytotic vesicles, mainly of the coated type, are frequently found along the neuronal plasma membrane in all developmental stages (Figs. 5, 6a, d, 20). As first suggested for other cells by Roth and Porter (1964), coated vesicles are specialized for the uptake of proteins. Nerve cells of the spinal ganglia can also take up proteins through pinocytosis (Rosenbluth and Wissig, 1964; Holtzman and Peterson, 1969), as nerve cells from other districts do (Brightman, 1965; Selwood, 1970). A part of the proteins taken up by the ganglionic nerve cells surely comes from the connective tissue space; however, the neuron might also take up proteins synthesized by the satellite cells.

Button-like, adhering junctions may be found at the neuron-satellite cell boundary (Fig. 22d) since satellite cells become detectable in the ganglion (Pannese, 1969; Tennyson, 1970b). Along the junction the apposed plasma membranes pursue a parallel, usually straight, course and are separated by a cleft, about 200 Å across, which is occupied by an apparently amorphous material of moderate density. A dense material is condensed in the cytoplasmic matrix on either side of the apposed plasma membranes. Adhering junctions are evident along the neuron-satellite cell boundary also during the successive developmental stages and in the adult (Fig. 22e) (Pannese, 1969; Tennyson, 1970b), as well as in the spiral (Adamo and Daigneault, 1972) and otic ganglia (Dixon, 1966) of adult animals. Apparently, occluding or gap junctions have never been described at the neuron-satellite cell boundary in spinal ganglia.

Junctions between nerve and neuroglial cells have been described in the last few years also in the sensitive corpuscles of Vertebrates and in the central nervous system of Invertebrates and Vertebrates. Junctions have been observed between nerve ending and inner bulb cells in the corpuscles of Herbst (Saxod, 1970; Halata, 1971) and in the bulbs of Krause (Spassova, 1971). In the central nervous system, junctions have been found between nerve and neuroglial cells in the leech (Gray and Guillery, 1963; Coggeshall and Fawcett, 1964), between giant axons and neuroglial cell processes in the earthworm (Coggeshall, 1965; Zimmermann, 1968), between axons and ependymal cells in guinea pigs (Wittkowski, 1967).

Junctions have been found also between axons and specialized neuroglial cells of the neurohypophysis in the eel (Knowles and Vollrath, 1965) and in guinea pigs (Wittkowski, 1967).

Whereas some of the junctions observed along the neuron-glial interface have been interpreted as devices for maintaining cohesion between adjacent cells, others have been identified as possible synapses. Pending physiological studies on this question, no conclusion on the significance of the junctions between nerve and satellite cells in the spinal ganglia may be drawn from the morphological studies hitherto performed.

As it is known, in the spinal ganglia several types of neurons have been described with the light microscope, some of these would have synaptic contacts on their bodies (see Scharf, 1958 for a review). However, as far as I know, electron microscopic evidence of synapses occurring *in vivo* on or among the spinal ganglion neurons has never been reported. The only electron microscopic evidence of synapses on the nerve cells of the spinal ganglia which I know of, has been found by Miller *et al.* (1970) in dissociated cell cultures from chick embryo spinal ganglia. These synapses, however, are probably *de novo* established *in vitro*.

4. Quantitative Relationship between Nerve and Satellite Cells (during Development)

A progressive increase in number of satellite cells takes place during ganglionic development. Satellite cells are less numerous than neuroblasts in stage *a*, but they outnumber nerve cells in stage *c*. The difference in number between satellite and nerve cells is even greater in the adult.

During developmental stages *a* and *b* the increase in number of satellite cells depends mainly on differentiation of undifferentiated cells, but later on (stage *c*) it seems due mainly to mitosis of fully differentiated satellite cells.

From stage *c* to the final developmental stage the nerve cells do no longer increase in number, although they increase gradually in volume. In this period each nerve cell is completely enveloped by a satellite cell sheath, which also increases gradually in volume. This increase in volume is certainly related to an increase in number of satellite cells; it has not been established whether it depends also on an increase in volume of each satellite cell. Therefore, during ganglionic development the satellite cell sheath enveloping a given nerve cell body adjusts its total mass to the increasing neuronal size. Through this adjustment, a quantitative balance between the satellite cell sheath and the related nerve cell body is reached at the end of development. In the spinal ganglia of adult animals, in fact, the volume of each satellite cell sheath is directly proportional both to the volume and to the surface area of the related nerve cell body (Pannese *et al.*, 1972).

This balance is probably important for the functional activity of the ganglionic nerve cell. In fact, if the satellite cells play a trophic role toward the related nerve cell by supporting the latter metabolically, the total mass of satellite cells per each ganglionic nerve cell is likely to depend on the volume and metabolic activity of the nerve cell.

Besides, the gradual increase in number of the satellite cells belonging to the same perineuronal sheath during ganglionic development makes the system of extracellular clefts formed by the overlapping of satellite cells gradually more extensive in each perineuronal sheath. Also this fact is probably significant as many materials coming from the blood vessels and interstitial spaces of the ganglion gain access to the surface of the nerve cell by passage through the mentioned system of clefts (Rosenbluth and Wissig, 1964; Villegas and Villegas, 1964; Baker, 1965; Holtzman and Peterson, 1969; Brown et al., 1969), which open at the surface of the perikaryon and in the light space (lamina lucida) under the basal lamina[3] respectively.

5. Development of the Ganglionic Interstitial Spaces

With the light microscope Brizzee (1949) observed that in the spinal ganglia of the chick embryo the fibroblasts are first evident between the 15th and 18th incubation day, that is much later than the satellite cells. The fibroblasts could penetrate the ganglion together with the connective tissue sheaths of the blood vessels.

More recently also the electron microscope has been used to study the formation of the ganglionic interstitial spaces in the chick embryo (Pannese, 1969). The following stages (a to d) have been recognized: each one of these stages unfolds in parallel to the stage of satellite cell development previously indicated with the same letter (see p. 60 to 62).

a) At this stage, i.e. when the satellite cells are first detectable, the ganglion still shows an epithelium-like structure (Figs. 20, 23), its cells (undifferentiated cells, neuroblasts, and satellite cells) being separated everywhere by clefts about 200 Å in width. A basal lamina covers the whole contour of the ganglion and neatly delimits it from the surrounding mesenchyme (Fig. 5). Sometimes fine fibrils can be found close to the outer limit of the basal lamina.

b) At this stage interstitial spaces first appear in the ganglion as intercellular clefts which are in some places widened locally or for some distance. Satellite cells usually border these primitive interstitial spaces (Figs. 8, 24a), but sometimes even undifferentiated cells and/or mitotic cells face them for a short distance. While the perikaryon of the neuroblasts never comes in direct contact with these spaces, naked neuroblastic processes sometimes project in them. The boundary between satellite cell and the primitive interstitial space is usually quite regular (Figs. 8, 24a), as the plasma membrane of the satellite cell exhibits a smooth or slightly wavy course. The primitive interstitial spaces usually contain patches ("interstitial bodies" of Low, 1970) of a moderately dense material (Figs. 8, 24a)

Fig. 23. Part of a spinal ganglion showing an epithelium-like structure (spinal ganglion of a chick embryo: 13500 ×). The cells are separated everywhere by clefts about 200 Å in width, interstitial spaces being still absent. The cell labeled N_1 is a primitive neuroblast at an advanced developmental stage. The cells labeled N_2 are intermediate neuroblasts. Arrow points to confronting subsurface cisternae in two adjacent neuroblasts

---

3 To avoid confusion, the thin layer of apparently amorphous material which encircles the whole ganglionic rudiment in early developmental stages and that successively follows the outer contour of the satellite cell sheaths is indicated in this paper with the term basal lamina proposed by Fawcett (1966), instead of the term basement membrane. In fact, the term basement membrane was originally employed by light microscopists to indicate a much thicker structure including also collagen fibrils.

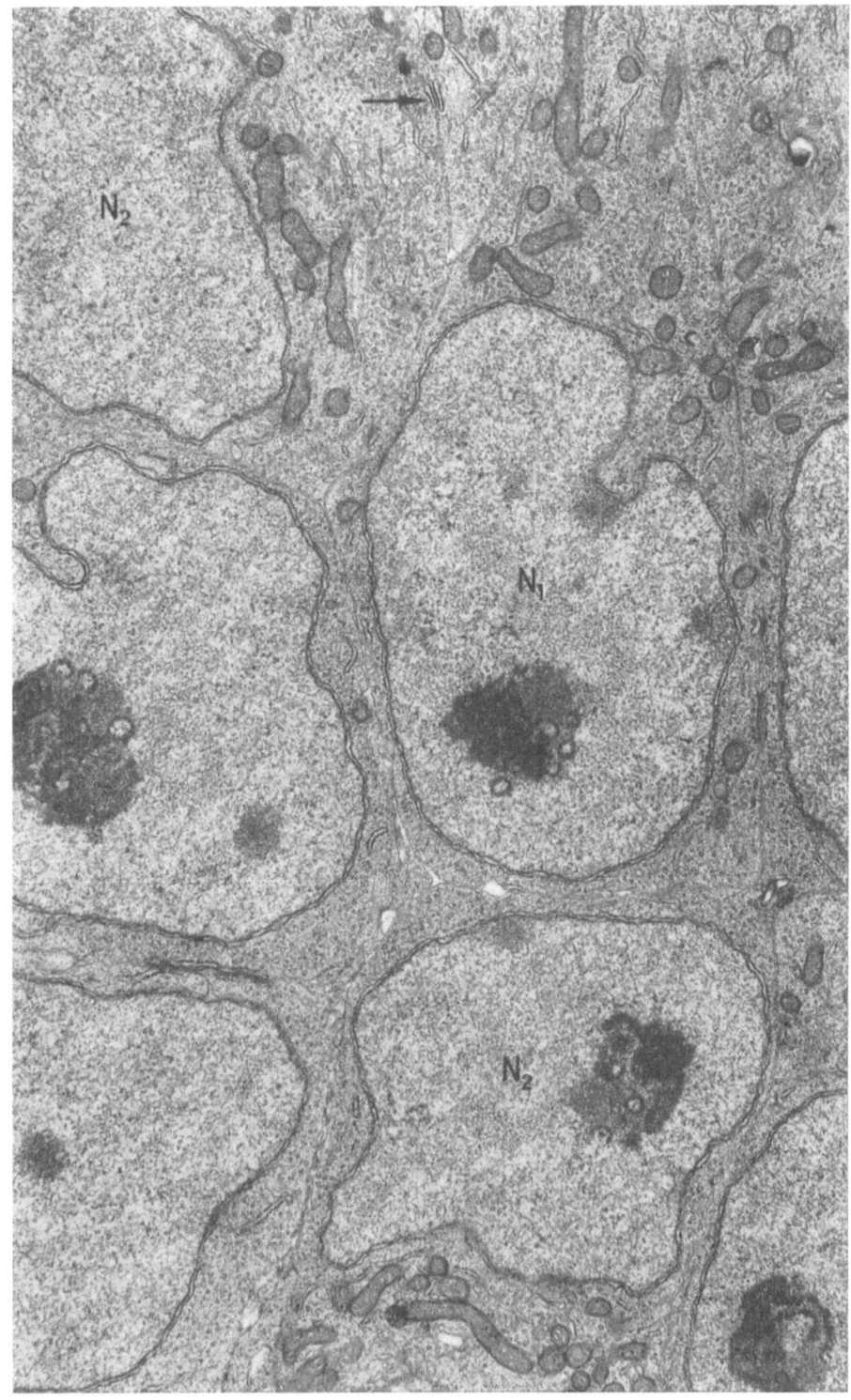

Fig. 23

which appears amorphous at low magnification. At higher magnification this material appears as a mat of thin filaments with scattered small granules. Sometimes the spaces also contain fibrils less than 100 Å thick, which can be individually scattered or arranged in fine bundles.

The seemingly amorphous material may lie near the plasma membrane of the cells facing the space (Figs. 8, 24a), thus forming a primordium of the basal lamina. This lamina, however, is never continuous but it always shows interruptions.

At present many evidences suggest that the basal lamina of epithelia is synthesized, at least in part, by the adjacent epithelial cells (Pierce jr. *et al.*, 1962, 1964; Hay and Revel, 1963; Pierce jr., 1964, 1966; Mukerjee *et al.*, 1965; Dodson, 1967; Briggaman *et al.*, 1971; Cohen and Hay, 1971; Dodson and Hay, 1971; Hay and Dodson, 1973). Instead, the origin of the basal lamina which follows the contour of satellite and Schwann cells is still a matter of speculations. Materials resembling those of the basal lamina have been found in the cytoplasmic matrix close to the outer surface in Schwann cells by Blümcke and Niedorf (1965). As to the satellite cells, Tennyson (1970b) maintains that they are responsible for the induction of their own basal lamina.

c) At this stage the interstitial spaces appear rather enlarged and they completely separate the satellite cell sheath related to a nerve cell from the sheaths enveloping neighboring nerve cells (Fig. 24b). As a consequence, at this stage each satellite cell appears related to one nerve cell only. Folds and finger-like projections arising from the satellite cells can protrude in the interstitial spaces; moreover, grooves can be observed along the outer contour of the satellite cell sheath. These projections and grooves render somewhat irregular the originally smooth boundary between the satellite cell sheath and the interstitial space.

An apparently amorphous material, fine fibrils (Fig. 24b), collagen fibrils of different thickness, and occasionally fibroblasts may be found in the interstitial spaces. Bundles of collagen fibrils are sometimes situated in grooves of the fibroblastic and of the satellite cells surface. Rarely a satellite cell completely encircles a bundle of collagen fibrils with its attenuated cytoplasmic expansions. The intimate relationship between satellite cells and collagen fibrils recalls that between fibroblasts and collagen fibrils observed in lymph nodes by Han (1961) and Clark (1962) and in the divided sciatic nerve by Morris *et al.* (1972). A similar relationship has also been observed between Schwann cells and collagen fibrils in peripheral nerves (Ochoa and Vial, 1967). Obviously, this relationship is not sufficient by itself to warrant the view that satellite cells are capable of producing collagen

Fig. 24a–c. Interstitial spaces. Fig. a (spinal ganglion of a chick embryo: 20000 ×) shows a primitive interstitial space containing a patch of moderately dense material (*). The interstitial space is bordered by satellite cells (*sc*) so that the perikarya of the neuroblasts N_1, N_2, and N_3 do not come in direct contact with it. Arrow points to a temporary junction, which links two satellite cells enveloping different neuroblasts (N_1 and N_3). Fig. b (spinal ganglion of a chick embryo: 20000 ×) shows an interstitial space containing fine fibrils, and patches of a moderately dense material. At arrow this material lies near the plasma membrane of a satellite cell, thus forming a primordium of the basal lamina. This interstitial space completely separates the satellite cells (*sc*) related to the neuroblast N_1 from those related to the neuroblast N_2. Fig. c (spinal ganglion of an adult rabbit: 10000 ×) shows the boundary between a satellite cell sheath (*sc*) and the interstitial space (*is*) at the end of body growth. This boundary is outlined in ink to show its complicated course. *f* fibrocytes, *nc* nerve cell

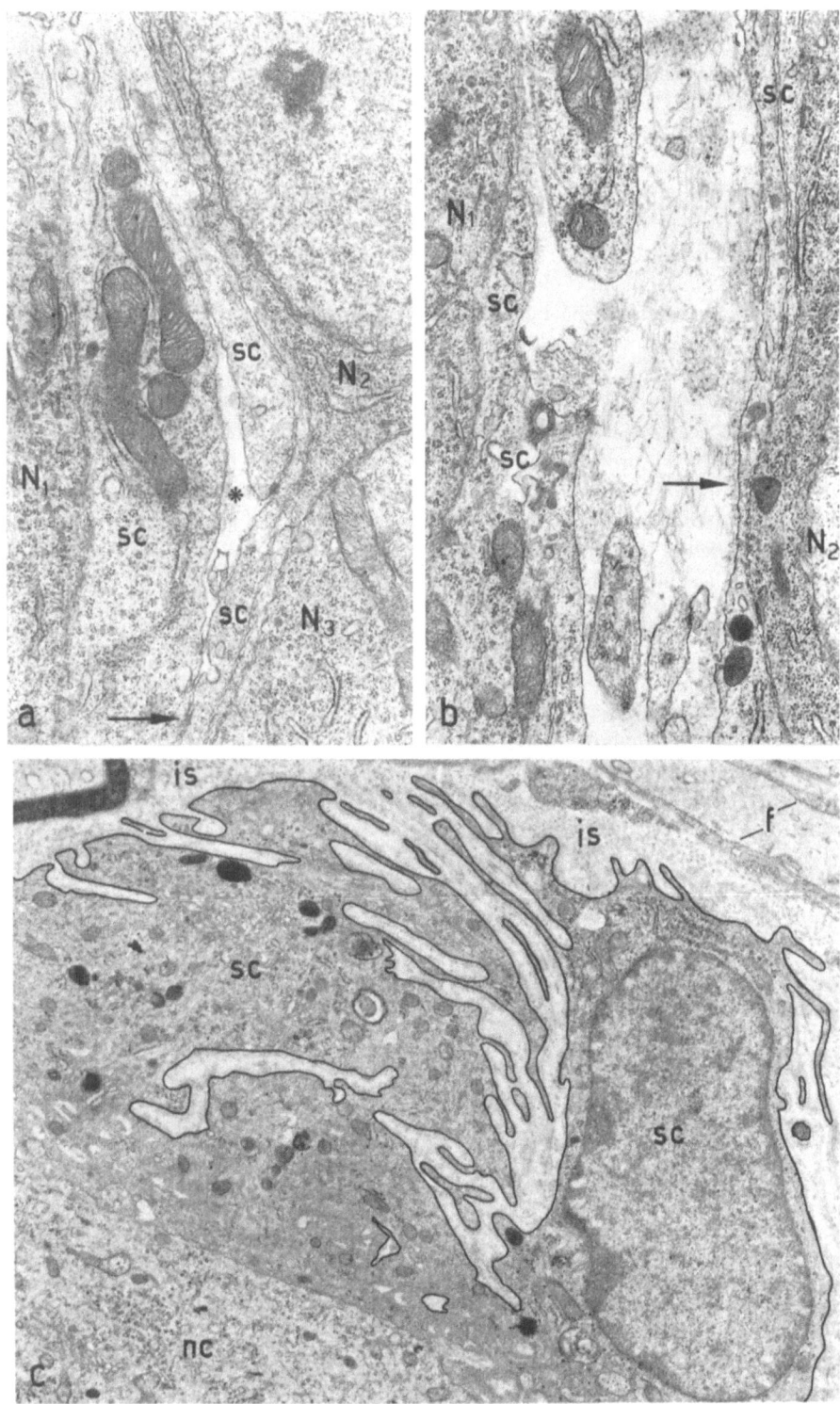

Fig. 24 a–c

as fibroblasts do. It may be only recalled that this suggestion has been advanced long ago for satellite cells by Levi (1908) and in recent years for both satellite and Schwann cells by Peterson and Murray (1960) and for the last cells by Causey (1960), Barton (1962), Nathaniel and Pease (1963) (see Thomas, 1964 for a discussion).

d) The interstitial spaces intervening between the satellite cell sheaths which belong to different neurons appear wider than during the preceding stage: they contain many collagen fibrils (Figs. 21, 22 b, 24 c) and some fibrocytes (Fig. 24 c). A continuous basal lamina completely covers the outer contour of the satellite cell sheath. This contour is characterized by many folds and finger-like projections and by numerous invaginations, which are sometimes deep and follow a complicated course within the satellite cell sheath (Figs. 22 b, 24 c). These invaginations contain an apparently amorphous material and, sometimes, also collagen fibrils. In this stage, therefore, the boundary between the satellite cell sheath and the interstitial space is usually very irregular (Figs. 21, 22 b, 24 c).

Sometimes the profile of a satellite cell projection arising from a satellite cell sheath at another level may appear isolated in the interstitial space; a basal lamina follows the contour of the satellite cell projection. This is a distinctive feature between satellite cell projections and cytoplasmic processes of the connective tissue cells, as the latter are devoid of a basal lamina (Fig. 25 b).

6. Development of Blood Vessels

When the ganglion still shows an epithelium-like structure, blood vessels have not entered the ganglion, while they are present in the mesenchyme surrounding the ganglion. In some cases the outer contour of these vessels is only 0.5μ from the basal lamina which covers the contour of the ganglion.

A few capillaries penetrate the ganglion after the appearance of the primitive interstitial spaces. The endothelial cells of the capillaries show a thick cytoplasm (Fig. 25 a) containing many free[4] polysomes, a few cisternae of the rough-surfaced endoplasmic reticulum, a Golgi complex, and mitochondria with a dense matrix. Many junctions link the endothelial cells.

The relationship between endothelial and neighboring cells of the ganglion may differ along the same capillary. In fact, a discontinuous cleft, containing a basal lamina, an apparently amorphous material (Fig. 25 a), and some fibrils surrounds the capillary wall. Where this interstice is not present, endothelial cells appear closely apposed to neighboring cells of the ganglion.

Fig. 25a and b. Blood vessels. Fig. a (spinal ganglion of a chick embryo: 18000 ×) shows a cross-section of a capillary which has presumably recently penetrated the ganglionic rudiment. In this section, a cleft containing an apparently amorphous material intervenes between endothelial and neighboring cells of the ganglion only at *. Elsewhere the endothelial cells come into direct contact with neighboring cells. *e* erythrocyte. Fig. b (spinal ganglion of a chick at hatching: 32000 ×) shows a portion of a capillary whose outer contour is covered by a basal lamina (*bl*). An interstitial space (*is*) containing an apparently amorphous material, collagen fibrils, and an attenuated expansion of a fibrocyte (*f*) intervenes between the capillary and the satellite cells (*sc*). *e* erythrocyte

4 See note on p. 10.

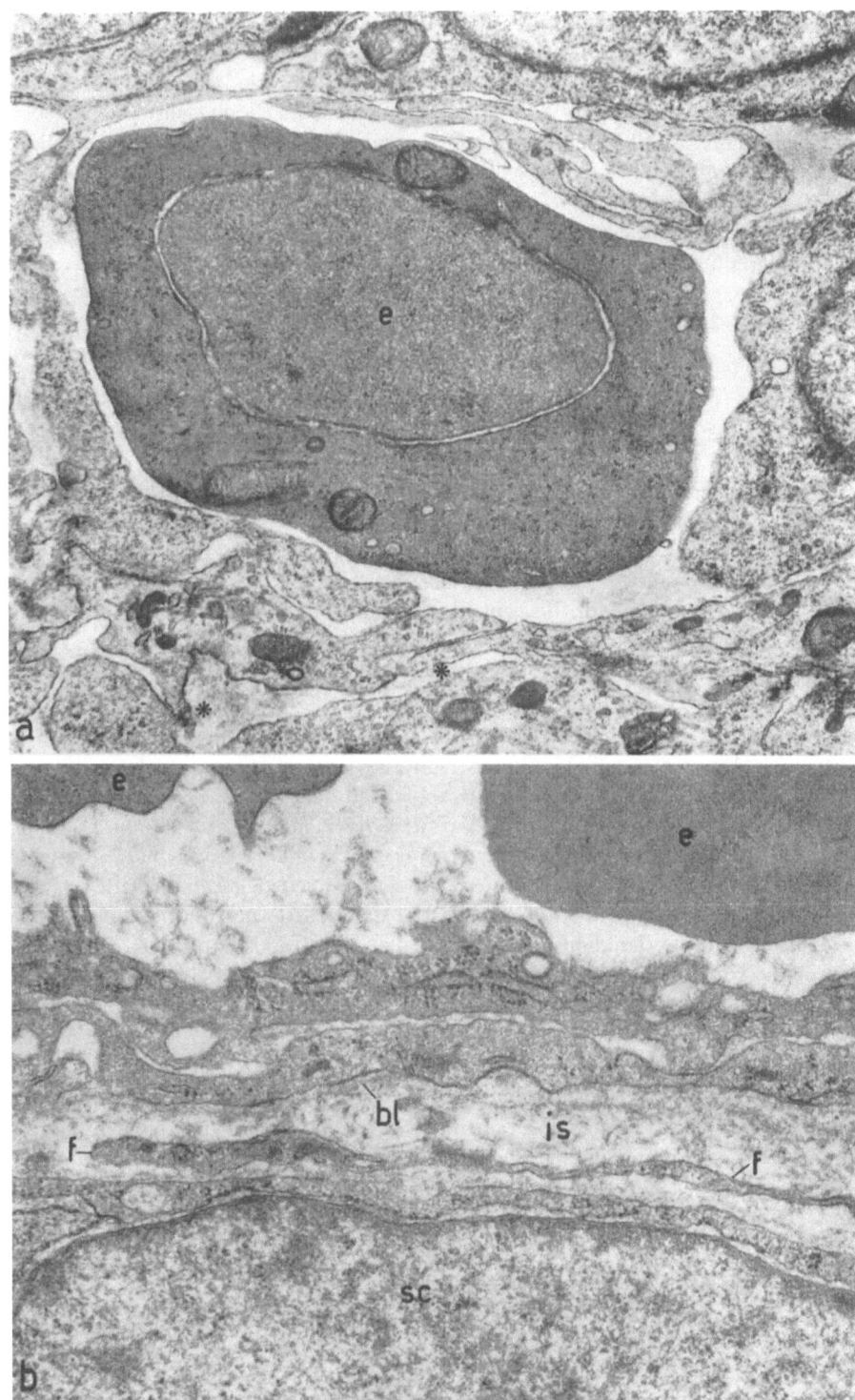

Fig. 25a and b

Later capillaries become more numerous within the ganglion. The cytoplasm of the endothelial cells appears attenuated in respect to the previous stage, and a continuous basal lamina covers the outer contour of the capillary everywhere (Fig. 25 b). The capillary is now surrounded by a continuous interstitial space containing collagen fibrils embedded in a moderately dense, apparently amorphous material: usually, attenuated expansions of fibroblasts or fibrocytes are also present in the pericapillary interstitial space (Fig. 25 b). Satellite cells always intervene between the space mentioned and the nerve cells. At this stage, the pericapillary interstitial spaces are continuous with the interstitial spaces intervening between the ganglionic units, each consisting of a nerve cell body enveloped by its own satellite cell sheath.

VII. Concluding Remarks

It can be seen from what has been reported in this review that our knowledge on the morphological events which characterize the differentiation of the spinal ganglion neuron is today fairly well advanced. The rather limited knowledge available at the end of the last century, received a considerable impulse at the beginning of this century thanks to the application of impregnation methods to the early embryo. During the last fifteen years the progress of our knowledge has been due above all to the results obtained from electron microscopical research.

Information, however, on the biochemical events which characterize the differentiation of the spinal ganglion neuron is comparatively much scarcer. Up to now, in fact, it has been possible to identify and quantitatively determine only a few chemical compounds in the developing neuron of the spinal ganglia. Several difficulties have delayed the progress of knowledge in this field. From the data of the chemical analysis of entire isolated ganglia it is often difficult to assess whether a given compound belongs to the one or another of the different cell populations of the ganglion, or to determine the exact proportions of a given compound for each cell type. On the other hand, technical difficulties have up to the present hindered the application of biochemical microanalysis to isolated neuroblasts. In turn, the histochemical studies with the electron microscope on embryonic material are only at the beginning. From the application of the latter technique interesting information on both the nerve and satellite cells can be expected in the near future. Histochemical research could be particularly fruitful in the study of the changes in chemical composition and enzymatic equipment which occur when nerve and satellite cells establish close morphological relationships, or in the analysis of the possible differences between the nerve cell when still in mutual contact with adjacent neurons and, respectively, the nerve cell completely isolated by the enveloping satellite cell sheath.

Little information is now available on the development of the interstitial spaces and blood vessels in spinal ganglia. For example, the role which satellite cells may play in the synthesis of the basal lamina that lines the outer contour of the satellite cell sheath, and in the production of collagen fibrils is unknown.

Also the degenerative events affecting many ganglionic cells in a period of the spinal ganglion development are insufficiently known. Probably such events represent a special case only of the widespread process of cellular degeneration which occurs during embryonic life. This particular topic has prompted much descriptive and experimental study recently, but many questions not yet resolved persist. As regards the spinal ganglia in particular, further research is needed to determine more precisely the nature of the cells undergoing degeneration, the structural details of the process, the endo- and/or extracellular mechanisms involved, the origin and characteristics of the cells concerned in the removal of the remnants of degenerated elements and, above all, the factors causing cell death during embryonic life.

Summary

The relevant aspects of the histogenesis of spinal ganglia are reviewed on the basis of the pertinent literature and of the author's research on chicken embryos.

Both ganglionic neurons and satellite cells take their origin from the neural crest; connective tissue cells and blood vessels arising from the surrounding mesenchyme enter into the ganglionic rudiment later.

In the early ganglionic rudiment, cells maintain for some time an undifferentiated appearance: they are rounded or polyhedral with a chromatin-rich nucleus and a cytoplasmic rim containing mainly free ribosomal clusters. Proliferation of these elements contributes to the increase in volume of the ganglion. Soon some of these cells differentiate into neuroblasts, later on others develop the characteristic features of the satellite cells.

Neuronal differentiation is characterized by biochemical and morphological events, biochemical changes usually preceding the morphological ones. The appearance of AChE activity is the best known of these biochemical events. Morphological differentiation entails changes in the cell shape, emission of two processes, and marked structural changes of the perikaryon, namely development of an elaborated endoplasmic reticulum with attached polysomes, gradual enlargement of the Golgi complex, conspicuous and rapid increment of the chondriome, and formation of numerous neurofilaments arranged in bundles. These structural changes are common to other types of differentiating neurons.

The nuclear envelope seems to play an important role in sensory neuron differentiation: in fact, it seems to be involved in the biosynthesis of membrane for the rough-surfaced endoplasmic reticulum, as well as for the Golgi complex and mitochondria. Synthesis of AChE seems to commence at the level of the nuclear envelope, and it spreads successively to the rough-surfaced endoplasmic reticulum when the latter gradually develops. Mitosis of ganglionic cells undergoing biochemical or morphological differentiation has been observed; this evidence shows that neuronal differentiation does not necessarily begin after the end of the parent cell division only. In the rudiments of spinal ganglia as well as in other districts of the developing nervous system, a number of cells undergo degeneration. This event appears to be one of the controlling factors of the size of the cell population in the ganglia.

In early developmental stages the ganglionic rudiment exhibits an epithelial-like structure and it is entirely enveloped by a thin basal lamina. Blood vessels of the surrounding mesenchyme have not yet entered the ganglion at this stage. Adhering and gap junctions link together adjacent cells and seem to play a significant role in maintaining the cell organization of the ganglion which still lacks a connective stroma. Besides gap junctions may represent sites of exchange between adjacent cells: in this case they could be instrumental in the unfolding of an equivalent differentiation of all the cells of a given group, or in the establishment of differences between the cells of a group.

Later on satellite cells become recognizable as star-shaped elements whose attenuated cytoplasmic expansions intervene between adjacent neuroblasts. At this stage the latter largely outnumber satellite cells. The junctions which in the preceding stage linked adjacent neuroblasts, disappear when development of the satellite cells commences.

In a still more advanced stage the satellite cells change their earlier star shape to the mature flattened shape and envelope each nerve cell; simultaneously interstitial spaces appear and a few capillaries enter the ganglion.

In much advanced stages of development each nerve cell appears completely enveloped by a satellite cell sheath, which is in turn entirely surrounded by an interstitial space. Beginning from this developmental stage and even more so in adult life, satellite cells outnumber nerve cells. During ganglionic development satellite cells increase progressively in number first through differentiation of undifferentiated cells, later on by mitosis of fully differentiated satellite cells.

During development the neuron-satellite cell boundary becomes gradually more irregular and complicated; thereby, this boundary increases much more than it would through the mere increase in volume of the nerve cell. Adhering junctions may be found at this boundary since satellite cells become recognizable in the ganglion. In the course of ganglionic development the satellite cell sheath enveloping a given nerve cell body adjusts its total mass to the increasing neuronal size. Thus a quantitative balance between the satellite cell sheath and the related nerve cell body is reached at the end of development.

Acknowledgements. The author wishes to thank Prof. R. Amprino for much useful comments and critical advice on this review, Drs. R. Bianchi, M. Gioia, and R. Ventura for the preparation of the list of references, Miss A. Bertolasi for drawing Figs. 1, 3, 14, and 16, and Miss R. Acace for typing the manuscript.

The researches of Pannese and Pannese *et al.* summarized in this review were supported by grants of the National Research Council (C. N. R.) Italy.

References

Ackerman, G. A.: Electron microscopy of the bursa of Fabricius of the embryonic chick with particular reference to the lympho-epithelial nodules. J. Cell Biol. **13**, 127–146 (1962).

Adamo, N. J., Daigneault, E. A.: Desmosome-like junctions in the spiral ganglia of cats. Amer. J. Anat. **135**, 141–146 (1972).

Afzelius, B. A.: Electron microscopy of Golgi elements in sea urchin eggs. Exp. Cell Res. **11**, 67–85 (1956).

André, J.: Contribution à la connaissance du chondriome. J. Ultrastruct. Res. Suppl. **3**, 1–185 (1962).

Aoki, A.: Temporary cell junctions in the developing human renal glomerulus. Develop. Biol. **15**, 156–164 (1967).

Arnold, J. M.: Fine structure of the development of the cephalopod lens. J. Ultrastruct. Res. **17**, 527–543 (1967).

Asbury, A. K.: Schwann cell proliferation in developing mouse sciatic nerve. A radioautographic study. J. Cell Biol. **34**, 735–743 (1967).

Bade, E. G.: Bildung von Mitochondrien in der regenerierenden Leber der Maus. Z. Zellforsch. **61**, 754–768 (1964).

Bahr, G. F., Zeitler, E.: Study of mitochondria in rat liver. J. Cell Biol. **15**, 489–501 (1962).

Baker, P. F.: A method for the location of extracellular space in crab nerve. J. Physiol. (Lond.) **180**, 439–447 (1965).

Balfour, F. M.: On the development of the spinal nerves in Elasmobranch fishes. Phil. Trans. B **166**, 175–195 (1876).

Balinsky, B. I., Devis, R. J.: Origin and differentiation of cytoplasmic structures in the oocytes of Xenopus laevis. Acta Embryol. Morph. exp. (Palermo) **6**, 55–108 (1963).

Barasa, A., Maccotta, V., Filogamo, G.: Etude au microscope électronique des prolongements, périphérique et central, des cellules de ganglions spinaux d'embryons de poulet cultivés in vitro. Bull. Ass. Anat., 55° Congr. (Nancy), p. 115–122 (1970).

Barbieri, M., Laschi, R., Rizzoli, C.: Osservazioni con il microscopio elettronico di ribosomi cristallizzati. Boll. Soc. ital. Biol. sper. **44**, 778–779 (1968).

Barbieri, M., Simonelli, L., Simoni, P., Maraldi, N. M.: Ribosome crystallization. II. Ultrastructural study on nuclear and cytoplasmic ribosome crystallization in hypothermic cell cultures. J. submicr. Cytol. **2**, 33–49 (1970).

Bardeen, C. R.: The growth and histogenesis of the cerebrospinal nerves in mammals. Amer. J. Anat. **2**, 231—257 (1903).

Barton, A. A.: An electron microscope study of degeneration and regeneration of nerve. Brain **85**, 799–808 (1962).

Beard, J.: The development of the peripheral nervous system of Vertebrates. Quart. J. micr. Sci. **29**, 153–227 (1889).

Beckwith, C. J.: Genesis of the plasma structure in the egg of Hydractinia esinata. J. Morph. **25**, 189–251 (1914).

Behnke, O., Moe, H.: An electron microscope study of mature and differentiating Paneth cells in the rat, especially of their endoplasmic reticulum and lysosomes. J. Cell Biol. **22**, 633–652 (1964).

Behnke, O., Zelander, T.: Filamentous substructure of microtubules of the marginal bundle of mammalian blood platelets. J. Ultrastruct. Res. **19**, 147–165 (1967).

Bell, P. R., Mühlethaler, K.: The degeneration and reappearance of mitochondria in the egg cells of a plant. J. Cell Biol. **20**, 235–248 (1964).

Bellairs, R.: Cell death in chick embryos as studied by electron microscopy. J. Anat. (Lond.) **95**, 54–60 (1961).

Belt, W. D.: The origin of adrenal cortical mitochondria and liposomes: a preliminary report. J. biophys. biochem. Cytol. **4**, 337—340 (1958).

Bennett, M. V. L., Trinkaus, J. P.: Electrical coupling between embryonic cells by way of extracellular space and specialized junctions. J. Cell Biol. **44**, 592–610 (1970).

Bennett, T., Cobb, J. L. S.: Studies on the avian gizzard: the development of the gizzard and its innervation. Z. Zellforsch. **98**, 599–621 (1969).

Berg, W. E., Humphreys, W. J.: Electron microscopy of four-cell stages of the ascidians Ciona and Styela. Develop. Biol. **2**, 42–60 (1960).

Berger, E. R.: Mitochondria genesis in the retinal photoreceptor inner segment. J. Ultrastruct. Res. **11**, 90–111 (1964).

Besta, C.: Sul modo di formazione della cellula nervosa nei gangli spinali del pollo. Riv. sper. Freniat. **30**, 133–134 (1904a).

Besta, C.: Ricerche intorno al modo con cui si stabiliscono i rapporti mutui tra gli elementi nervosi embrionali e sulla formazione del reticolo interno della cellula nervosa. Riv. sper. Freniat. **30**, 633–647 (1904b).

Bidder, F., Küpffer, C.: Untersuchungen über die Textur des Rückenmarkes und die Entwickelung seiner Formelemente. Leipzig 1857.

Biervliet, J. van: La substance chromophile pendant le cours du développement de la cellule nerveuse (Chromolyse physiologique et chromolyse expérimentale). Névraxe **1**, 33–55 (1900).

Bikle, D., Tilney, L. G., Porter, K. R.: Microtubules and pigment migration in the melano-phores of Fundulus heteroclitus L. Protoplasma (Wien) **61**, 322–345 (1966).

Billings, S. M.: Development of the Mauthner cell in Xenopus laevis: a light and electron microscopic study of the perikaryon. Z. Anat. Entwickl.-Gesch. **136**, 168–191 (1972).

Birks, R. I., Weldon, P. R.: Formation of crystalline ribosomal arrays in cultured chick embryo dorsal root ganglia. J. Anat. (Lond.) **109**, 143–156 (1971).

Blümcke, S., Niedorf, H. R.: Elektronenmikroskopischer Beitrag zur Bildung der Basalmembran Schwannscher Zellen. Naturwissenschaften **52**, 621 (1965).

Bodian, D.: Development of fine structure of spinal cord in monkey fetuses. I. The moto-neuron neuropil at the time of onset of reflex activity. Bull. Johns Hopk. Hosp. **119**, 129–149 (1966).

Bodian, D.: Development of fine structure of spinal cord in monkey fetuses. II. Pre-reflex period to period of long intersegmental reflexes. J. comp. Neurol. **133**, 113–166 (1968).

Bouck, G. B.: Fine structure and organelle associations in brown algae. J. Cell Biol. **26**, 523–537 (1965).

Bouck, G. B., Brown, D. L.: Microtubule genesis and cell shape in Ochromonas. J. Cell Biol. **47**, 22A–23A (1970).

Brandt, P. W., Pappas, G. D.: Mitochondria. II. The nuclear-mitochondrial relationship in Pelomyxa carolinensis Wilson (Chaos chaos L.). J. biophys. biochem. Cytol. **6**, 91–96 (1959).

Breemen, V. L. van: Neurofilaments as a model of the fundamental protoplasmic skeleton. Anat. Rec. **142**, 345 (1962).

Bremer, F.: Some problems in neurophysiology. London: Athlone Press 1953.

Briggaman, R. A., Dalldorf, F. G., Wheeler, C. E., Jr.: Formation and origin of basal lamina and anchoring fibrils in adult human skin. J. Cell Biol. **51**, 384–395 (1971).

Brightman, M. W.: The distribution within the brain of ferritin injected into cerebrospinal fluid compartments. II. Parenchymal distribution. Amer. J. Anat. **117**, 193—219 (1965).

Brightman, M. W., Reese, T. S.: Junctions between intimately apposed cell membranes in the vertebrate brain. J. Cell Biol. **40**, 648–677 (1969).

Brizzee, K. R.: Histogenesis of the supporting tissue in the spinal and the sympathetic trunk ganglia in the chick. J. comp. Neurol. **91**, 129–146 (1949).

Brown, D. A., Stumpf, W. E., Roth, L. J.: Location of radioactively labelled extracellular fluid indicators in nervous tissue by autoradiography. J. Cell Sci. **4**, 265–288 (1969).

Bunge, M. B.: Fine structure of nerve fibers and growth cones of isolated sympathetic neurons in culture. J. Cell Biol. **56**, 713–735 (1973).

Bunge, M. B., Bunge, R. P., Peterson, E. R., Murray, M. R.: A light and electron microscope study of long-term organized cultures of rat dorsal root ganglia. J. Cell Biol. **32**, 439–466 (1967).

Burn, J. H., Rand, M. J.: Sympathetic postganglionic mechanism. Nature (Lond.) **184**, 163–165 (1959).

Burn, J. H., Rand, M. J.: Acetylcholine in adrenergic transmission. Ann. Rev. Pharmacol. **5**, 163–182 (1965).

Buvat, R.: Sur la néoformation de mitochondries à partir du phragmoplaste, dans le méri-stème radiculaire du Blé. C. R. Acad. Sci. (Paris) **248**, 1014–1017 (1959).

Buvat, R.: Electron microscopy of plant protoplasm. Int. Rev. Cytol. **14**, 41–155 (1963).

Byers, B.: Ribosome crystallization induced in chick embryo tissues by hypothermia. J. Cell Biol. **30**, C1–C6 (1966).

Byers, B.: Structure and formation of ribosome crystals in hypothermic chick embryo cells. J. molec. Biol. **26**, 155–167 (1967).

Byers, B., Porter, K. R.: Oriented microtubules in elongating cells of the developing lens rudiment after induction. Proc. nat. Acad. Sci. (Wash.) **52**, 1091–1099 (1964).

Cajal, S. Ramón y: Sur l'origine et les ramifications des fibres nerveuses de la moelle embryon-naire. Anat. Anz. **5**, 85–95 (1890a).

Cajal, S. Ramón y: A quelle époque apparaissent les expansions des cellules nerveuses de la moëlle épinière du poulet? Anat. Anz. **5**, 609–613 (1890b).

Cajal, S. Ramón y: Estructura y conexiones de los ganglios simpaticos. Pequenas contri-buciones al conocimiento de los centros nerviosos de los vertebrados, p. 11. Barcelona 1891.

Cajal, S. Ramón y: Asociacion del método del nitrato de plata con el embrionario. Para el estudio de los focos motores y sensitivos. Trab. Lab. Invest. Biol. Univ. Madrid 3, 65–96 (1904).

Cajal, S. Ramón y: Histologie du système nerveux de l'homme et des vertébrés, vol. 1. Paris: Maloine 1909.

Caley, D. W., Maxwell, D. S.: An electron microscopic study of neurons during postnatal development of the rat cerebral cortex. J. comp. Neurol. 133, 17–44 (1968).

Campbell, G. Le M., Weintraub, H., Mayall, B. H., Holtzer, H.: Primitive erythropoiesis in early chick embryo-genesis. II. Correlation between hemoglobin synthesis and the mitotic history. J. Cell Biol. 50, 669–681 (1971).

Carasso, N., Favard, P.: L'appareil de Golgi. In: Traité de microscopie électronique, edit. C. Magnan, vol. 2, p. 963–997. Paris: Hermann 1961.

Cassidy, M. M., Tidball, C. S.: Cellular mechanism of intestinal permeability alterations produced by chelation depletion. J. Cell Biol. 32, 685–698 (1967).

Causey, G.: The cell of Schwann. Edinburgh and London: E. & S. Livingstone Ltd. 1960.

Chèvremont, M.: Etude des chondriosomes par la microscopie et la microcinematographie en contraste de phase. Monit. zool. ital. 61 Suppl., 127–130 (1953).

Chrétien, M.: Formation de nouveaux appareils de Golgi dans des cellules secrétrices soumises à une stimulation hormonale. J. Microscopie 11, 39–40 (1971).

Clark, S.L., Jr.: The reticulum of lymph nodes in mice studied with the electron microscope. Amer. J. Anat. 110, 217–257 (1962).

Cloney, R. A.: Cytoplasmic filaments and cell movements: epidermal cells during ascidian metamorphosis. J. Ultrastruct. Res. 14, 300–328 (1966).

Clouet, D. H., Waelsch, H.: Amino acid and protein metabolism of the brain. VIII. The recovery of cholinesterase in the nervous system of the frog after inhibition. J. Neurochem. 8, 201–215 (1961).

Clowes, F. A. L., Juniper, B. E.: The fine structure of the quiescent center and neighbouring tissues in root meristems. J. exp. Bot. 15, 622–630 (1964).

Cobb, J. L. S., Bennett, T.: An ultrastructural study of mitotic division in differentiated gastric smooth muscle cells. Z. Zellforsch. 108, 177–189 (1970).

Coggeshall, R. E.: A fine structural analysis of the ventral nerve cord and associated sheath of Lumbricus terrestris L. J. comp. Neurol. 125, 393–438 (1965).

Coggeshall, R. E., Fawcett, D. W.: The fine structure of the central nervous system of the leech, Hirudo medicinalis. J. Neurophysiol. 27, 229–289 (1964).

Cohen, A. M., Hay, E. D.: Secretion of collagen by embryonic neuroepithelium at the time of spinal cord-somite interaction. Develop. Biol. 26, 578–605 (1971).

Collin, R.: Recherches cytologiques sur le développement de la cellule nerveuse. Névraxe 8, 185–309 (1906).

Conradi, S.: Ultrastructural specialization of the initial axon segment of cat lumbar motoneurons. Acta Soc. Med. upsalien. 71, 281–284 (1966).

Cossel, L.: Die menschliche Leber im Elektronenmikroskop. Jena: VEB Gustav Fischer 1964.

Crain, S. M., Benitez, H., Vatter, A. E.: Some cytologic effects of salivary nerve-growth factor on tissue cultures of peripheral ganglia. In: Symposium on the nerve growth factor, edit. H. E. Whipple. Ann. N. Y. Acad. Sci. 118, 206–231 (1964).

Cravioto, H.: The role of Schwann cells in the development of human peripheral nerves. An electron microscopic study. J. Ultrastruct. Res. 12, 634–651 (1965).

Dahlström, A.: Effects of vinblastine and colchicine on monoamine containing neurons of the rat, with special regard to the axoplasmic transport of amine granules. Acta neuropath. (Berl.) Suppl. 5, 226–237 (1971).

Dallner, G., Siekevitz, P., Palade, G. E.: Biogenesis of endoplasmic reticulum membranes. I. Structural and chemical differentiation in developing rat hepatocyte. J. Cell Biol. 30, 73–96 (1966).

Dalton, A. J.: Golgi apparatus and secretion granules. In: The cell, edit. J. Brachet and A. E. Mirsky, vol. 2, p. 603–619. New York and London: Academic Press 1961.

Daniels, E. W.: Origin of the Golgi system in amoebae. Z. Zellforsch. 64, 38–51 (1964).

Daniels, M. P.: Colchicine inhibition of nerve fiber formation in vitro. J. Cell Biol. 53, 164–176 (1972).

David, H.: Zur Mitochondrienneubildung in den Leberzellen des Feuersalamanders (Sala-
mandra maculata). Z. Zellforsch. **57**, 567–571 (1962).

Davison, P. F., Huneeus, F. C.: Fibrillar proteins from squid axons. II. Microtubule protein.
J. molec. Biol. **52**, 429–439 (1970).

DeHaan, R. L.: Regulation of spontaneous activity and growth of embryonic chick heart
cells in tissue culture. Develop. Biol. **16**, 216–249 (1967).

Del Cerro, M. P., Snider, R. S.: Studies on the developing cerebellum. Ultrastructure of the
growth cones. J. comp. Neurol. **133**, 341–362 (1968).

De Petris, S., Karlsbad, G.: Localization of antibodies by electron microscopy in developing
antibody-producing cells. J. Cell Biol. **26**, 759–778 (1965).

De Robertis, E., Bleichmar, H.: Mitochondriogenesis in nerve fibers of the infrared receptor
membrane of pit vipers. Z. Zellforsch. **57**, 572–582 (1962).

De-Thé, G.: Cytoplasmic microtubules in different animal cells. J. Cell Biol. **23**, 265–275
(1964).

Detwiler, S. R.: An experimental study of spinal nerve segmentation in Amblystoma with
reference to the plurisegmental contribution to the brachial plexus. J. exp. Zool. **67**,
395–441 (1934).

Detwiler, S. R.: Application of vital dyes to the study of sheath cell origin. Proc. Soc. exp.
Biol. (N. Y.) **37**, 380–382 (1937).

Diers, L.: On the plastids, mitochondria, and other cell constituents during oögenesis of a
plant. J. Cell Biol. **28**, 527–543 (1966).

Diner, O.: Les cellules de Schwann en mitose et leurs rapports avec les axones au cours du
développement du nerf sciatique chez le rat. C. R. Acad. Sci. (Paris) **261**, 1731–1734
(1965).

Dixon, J. S.: The fine structure of parasympathetic nerve cells in the otic ganglia of the
rabbit. Anat. Rec. **156**, 239–251 (1966).

Dodson, J. W.: The differentiation of epidermis. I. The interrelationship of epidermis and
dermis in embryonic chicken skin. J. Embryol. exp. Morph. **17**, 83–105 (1967).

Dodson, J. W., Hay, E. D.: Secretion of collagenous stroma by isolated epithelium grown *in
vitro*. Exp. Cell Res. **65**, 215–220 (1971).

Dohrn, A.: Nervenfaser und Ganglienzelle. Histogenetische Untersuchungen. Mittheil. Zool.
Station Neapel **10**, 255–341 (1891).

Donaldson, H. H., Nagasaka, G.: On the increase in the diameters of nerve cell bodies and
of the fibers arising from them-during the later phases of growth (albino rat). J. comp.
Neurol. **29**, 529–552 (1918).

Droz, B.: Synthèse et transfert des protéines cellulaires dans les neurones ganglionnaires;
étude radioautographique quantitative en microscopie électronique. J. Microscopie **6**,
201–228 (1967).

Droz, B., Leblond, C. P.: Axonal migration of proteins in the central nervous system and
peripheral nerves as shown by radioautography. J. comp. Neurol. **121**, 325–346 (1963).

Dubois, P.: Origine et développement de l'appareil de Golgi au cours de la différenciation
cellulaire dans une glande endocrine chez l'homme: l'antéhypophyse foetale. J. Microscopie
13, 193–206 (1972).

DuShane, G. P.: Neural fold derivatives in the Amphibia: pigment cells, spinal ganglia and
Rohon-Beard cells. J. exp. Zool. **78**, 485–503 (1938).

Dvořák, M.: A contribution to the investigation of the role of the nuclear membrane in the
formation of endoplasmic reticulum. Folia morph. (Prague) **16**, 286–293 (1968).

Eccles, J. C.: Conduction and synaptic transmission in the nervous system. Ann. Rev. Physiol.
10, 93–116 (1948).

Ekholm, R., Hydén, H.: Polysomes from microdissected fresh neurons. J. Ultrastruct. Res.
13, 269–280 (1965).

Elliott, A. M., Bak, I. J.: The fate of mitochondria during aging in Tetrahymena pyriformis.
J. Cell Biol. **20**, 113–129 (1964).

England, J. M., Kadin, M. E., Goldstein, M. N.: The effect of vincristine sulphate on the axoplasmic flow of proteins in cultured sympathetic neurons. J. Cell Sci. **12**, 549–565 (1973).

Eränkö, O.: Histochemistry of nervous tissues: catecholamines and cholinesterases. Ann.
Rev. Pharmacol. **7**, 203–222 (1967).

Eränkö, O., Härkönen, M.: Effect of axon division on the distribution of noradrenaline and acetylcholinesterase in sympathetic neurons of the rat. Acta physiol. scand. 63, 411–412 (1965).

Eränkö, O., Härkönen, M., Kokko, A., Räisänen, L.: Histochemical and starch gel electrophoretic characterization of desmo- and lyo-esterases in the sympathetic and spinal ganglia of the rat. J. Histochem. Cytochem. 12, 570–581 (1964).

Ernst, M.: Über Untergang von Zellen während der normalen Entwicklung bei Wirbeltieren. Z. Anat. Entwickl.-Gesch. 79, 228–262 (1926).

Essner, E., Novikoff, A. B.: Acid phosphatase activity in hepatic lysosomes: electron microscopic demonstration of its reaction product. J. Histochem. Cytochem. 8, 318 (1960).

Essner, E., Novikoff, A. B.: Localization of acid phosphatase activity in hepatic lysosomes by means of electron microscopy. J. biophys. biochem. Cytol. 9, 773–784 (1961).

Essner, E., Novikoff, A. B.: Cytological studies on two functional hepatomas. J. Cell Biol. 15, 289–312 (1962).

Estable, C., Acosta-Ferreira, W., Sotelo, J. R.: An electron microscope study of the regenerating nerve fibers. Z. Zellforsch. 46, 387–399 (1957).

Falk, H., Kleinig, H.: Feinbau und Carotinoide von Tribonema (Xanthophyceae). Arch. Mikrobiol. 61, 347–362 (1968).

Famiglietti, E. V., Jr., Peters, A.: The synaptic glomerulus and the intrinsic neuron in the dorsal lateral geniculate nucleus of the cat. J. comp. Neurol. 144, 285–334 (1972).

Fauré-Fremiet, E., Favard, P., Carasso, N.: Étude au microscope électronique des ultrastructures d'Epistylis anastatica (Cilié Péritriche). J. Microscopie 1, 287–312 (1962).

Fawcett, D. W.: Observations on the cytology and electron microscopy of hepatic cells. J. nat. Cancer Inst. 15 Suppl., 1475–1502 (1955).

Fawcett, D. W.: The cell its organelles and inclusions. Philadelphia and London: W. B. Saunders Co. 1966.

Fawcett, D. W., McNutt, N. S.: The ultrastructure of the cat myocardium. I. Ventricular papillary muscle. J. Cell Biol. 42, 1–45 (1969).

Feldberg, W. S.: Transmission in the central nervous system and sensory transmission. Central and sensory transmission. Pharmacol. Rev. 6, 85–93 (1954).

Feldberg, W. S.: Acetylcholine. In: Metabolism of the nervous system, edit. D. Richter, p. 493–510. London-New York-Paris-Los Angeles: Pergamon Press 1957.

Fernandez, H. L., Huneeus, F. C., Davison, P. F.: Studies on the mechanism of axoplasmic transport in the crayfish cord. J. Neurobiol. 1, 395–409 (1970).

Ferreira, J. F. D.: A diferenciaçâo do condrioma aparelho de Golgi e ergastoplasma. Lisboa: Ramos, Alfonso & Moita, LDA 1959.

Filogamo, G.: Recherches expérimentales sur l'activité des cholinestérases spécifique et non spécifique, dans le développement du lobe optique du poulet. Arch. Biol. (Liège) 71, 159–198 (1960).

Fletcher, M. J., Sanadi, D. R.: Turnover of rat liver mitochondria. Biochem. biophys. Acta (Amst.) 51, 356–360 (1961).

Flickinger, C. J.: The development of Golgi complexes and their dependence upon the nucleus in amebae. J. Cell Biol. 43, 250–262 (1969).

Frederic, J.: Recherches cytologiques sur le chondriome normal ou soumis à l'expérimentation dans des cellules vivantes cultivées in vitro. Arch. Biol. (Liège) 69, 167–349 (1958).

Fujita, H., Fujita, S.: Electron microscopic studies on neuroblast differentiation in the central nervous system of domestic fowl. Z. Zellforsch. 60, 463–478 (1963).

Fukuda, T., Koelle, G. B.: The cytological localization of intracellular neuronal acetylcholinesterase. J. biophys. biochem. Cytol. 5, 433–440 (1959).

Gatenby, J. B.: The gametogenesis and early development of Limnaea stagnalis L., with special reference to the Golgi apparatus and mitochondria. Quart. J. micr. Sci. 63, 445–492 (1919).

Gatenby, J. B.: Notes on the gametogenesis of a pulmonate Mollusc. An electron microscope study. Cellule 60, 289–303 (1960).

Gay, H.: Chromosome-nuclear membrane-cytoplasmic interrelations in Drosophila. J. biophys. biochem. Cytol. 2 Suppl., 407–414 (1956).

Gerebtzoff, M. A.: Cholinestérases. London: Pergamon Press 1959.

Geren, B. B., Schmitt, F. O.: The structure of the Schwann cell and its relation to the axon in certain invertebrate nerve fibers. Proc. nat. Acad. Sci. (Wash.) 40, 863–870 (1954).

Gey, G. O., Shapras, P., Bang, F. B., Gey, M. K.: Some relations of inclusion droplets (pinocytosis, Lewis) and mitochondrial behavior in normal and malignant cells. In: Fine structure of cells, p. 38–54. Groningen: P. Noordhoff 1955.

Ghiara, G., Taddei, C., Filosa, S.: Un particolare tipo di costituente ribonucleoproteico del citoplasma di cellule follicolari e di ovociti in accrescimento di Lacerta s. sicula Raf. Acta med. romana 4, 59–67 (1966).

Giacobini, G., Marchisio, P. C., Giacobini, E., Koslow, S. H.: Developmental changes of cholinesterases and monoamine oxidase in chick embryo spinal and sympathetic ganglia. J. Neurochem. 17, 1177–1185 (1970).

Glücksmann, A.: Über die Entwicklung der quergestreiften Muskulatur und ihre funktionellen Beziehungen zum Skelet in der Onto- und Phylogenie der Wirbeltiere. Z. Anat. Entwickl.-Gesch. 103, 303–370 (1934).

Glücksmann, A.: Cell deaths in normal vertebrate ontogeny. Biol. Rev. 26, 59–86 (1951).

Goldman, R. D.: The role of three cytoplasmic fibers in BHK-21 cell motility. I. Microtubules and the effects of colchicine. J. Cell Biol. 51, 752–762 (1971).

Goldsmith, M., Weston, J. A., Cowell, L.: Crystalline bodies associated with morphogenetic cell death in embryonic sensory ganglia. Amer. Zool. 7, 755 (1967).

Golgi, C.: De nouveau sur la structure des cellules nerveuses des ganglions spinaux. Arch. ital. Biol. 31, 273–280 (1899).

Gonatas, N. K., Robbins, E.: The homology of spindle tubules and neurotubules in the chick embryo retina. Protoplasma (Wien) 59, 377–391 (1964).

Graham, M. A.: Sex chromatin in cell nuclei of the cat from the early embryo to maturity. Anat. Rec. 119, 469–491 (1954).

Grassé, P. P.: Ultrastructure, polarité et reproduction de l'appareil de Golgi. C. R. Acad. Sci. (Paris) 245, 1278–1281 (1957).

Gray, E. G., Guillery, R. W.: An electron microscopical study of the ventral nerve cord of the leech. Z. Zellforsch. 60, 826–849 (1963).

Gray, J.: The properties of an intercellular matrix and its relation to electrolytes. Brit. J. exp. Biol. 3, 167–187 (1926).

Grimstone, A. V.: Cytoplasmic membranes and the nuclear membrane in the flagellate Trichonympha. J. biophys. biochem. Cytol. 6, 369–378 (1959).

Gross, P. R., Philpott, D. E., Nass, S.: Electron microscopy of the centrifuged sea urchin egg, with a note on the structure of the ground cytoplasm. J. biophys. biochem. Cytol. 7, 135–142 (1960).

Halata, Z.: Die Ultrastruktur der Lamellenkörperchen bei Wasservögeln (Herbstsche Endigungen). Acta anat. (Basel) 80, 362–376 (1971).

Hamburger, V.: Experimental analysis of the dual origin of the trigeminal ganglion in the chick embryo. J. exp. Zool. 147, 91–123 (1961).

Hamburger, V.: Ontogeny of behaviour and its structural basis. In: Comparative neurochemistry, edit. D. Richter, p. 21–34. Oxford-London-New York-Paris: Pergamon Press 1964.

Hamburger, V., Balaban, M.: Observations and experiments on spontaneous rhythmical behavior in the chick embryo. Develop. Biol. 7, 533–545 (1963).

Hamburger, V., Levi-Montalcini, R.: Proliferation, differentiation and degeneration in the spinal ganglia of the chick embryo under normal and experimental conditions. J. exp. Zool. 111, 457–501 (1949).

Han, S. S.: The ultrastructure of the mesenteric lymph node of the rat. Amer. J. Anat. 109, 183–225 (1961).

Harrison, R. G.: Über die Histogenese des peripheren Nervensystems bei Salmo salar. Arch. mikr. Anat. 57, 354–444 (1901).

Harrison, R. G.: Neue Versuche und Beobachtungen über die Entwicklung der peripheren Nerven der Wirbeltiere. Sitzungsber. d. niederrhein. Ges. f. Natur u. Heilkunde, 55–62 (1904).

Harrison, R. G.: Observations on the living developing nerve fiber. Anat. Rec. 1, 116–118 (1907).

Harrison, R. G.: The outgrowth of the nerve fiber as a mode of protoplasmic movement. J. exp. Zool. **9**, 787–846 (1910).

Harrison, R. G.: Neuroblast versus sheath cell in the development of peripheral nerves. J. comp. Neurol. **37**, 123–205 (1924).

Harvey, E. B.: Structure and development of the clear quarter of the Arbacia punctulata egg. J. exp. Zool. **102**, 253–275 (1946).

Hatai, S.: A note on the significance of the form and contents of the nucleus in the spinal ganglion cells of the foetal rat. J. comp. Neurol. **14**, 27–48 (1904).

Hawley, E. S., Wagner, R. P.: Synchronous mitochondrial division in Neurospora crassa. J. Cell Biol. **35**, 489–499 (1967).

Hay, D. A., Low, F. N.: The fine structure of progressive stages of myocardial mitosis in chick embryos. Amer. J. Anat. **134**, 175–202 (1972).

Hay, E. D.: The fine structure of blastema cells and differentiating cartilage cells in regenerating limbs of Amblystoma larvae. J. biophys. biochem. Cytol. **4**, 583–592 (1958).

Hay, E. D.: Organization and fine structure of epithelium and mesenchyme in the developing chick embryo. In: Epithelial-mesenchymal interactions, edit. Fleischmajer, **p. 31–55**. Baltimore: Williams & Wilkins Co. 1968.

Hay, E. D., Dodson, J. W.: Secretion of collagen by corneal epithelium. I. Morphology of the collagenous products produced by isolated epithelia grown on frozen-killed lens. J. Cell Biol. **57**, 190–213 (1973).

Hay, E. D., Revel, J. P.: Autoradiographic studies of the origin of the basement lamella in Ambystoma. Develop. Biol. **7**, 152–168 (1963).

Hays, R. M., Singer, B., Malamed, S.: The effect of calcium withdrawal on the structure and function of the toad bladder. J. Cell Biol. **25**, 195–208 (1965).

Held, H.: Die Entstehung der Neurofibrillen. Neurol. Zbl. **24**, 706–710 (1905).

Held, H.: Zur Histogenese der Nervenleitung. Anat. Anz. Erg.-H. zu **29**, 185–205 (1906).

Held, H.: Die Entwicklung des Nervengewebes bei den Wirbeltieren. Leipzig: J. A. Barth 1909.

Herbst, C.: Über das Auseinandergehen von Furchungs und Gewebezellen in kalkfreiem Medium. Wilhelm Roux' Arch. Entwickl.-Mech. Org. **9**, 424–463 (1900).

Hett, J.: Histogenetische Untersuchungen über die menschliche Nebenniere. Anat. Anz. Erg.-H. zu **60**, 88–95 (1925).

Hinds, J. W., Ruffett, T. L.: Cell proliferation in the neural tube: an electron microscopic and Golgi analysis in the mouse cerebral vesicle. Z. Zellforsch. **115**, 226–264 (1971).

His, W.: Untersuchungen über die erste Anlage des Wirbelthierleibes. Die erste Entwickelung des Hühnchens im Ei. Leipzig 1868.

His, W.: Zur Geschichte des menschlichen Rückenmarkes und der Nervenwurzeln. Abh. math.-phys. Kl. d. Kgl. Sächs. Ges. Wiss. **13**, 479–513 (1886).

His, W.: Die Entwickelung der ersten Nervenbahnen beim menschlichen Embryo. Übersichtliche Darstellung. Arch. Anat. u. Physiol., Anat. Abt., 368–378 (1887).

His, W.: Histogenese und Zusammenhang der Nervenelemente. Arch. Anat. u. Physiol., Anat. Abt., Suppl., 95–117 (1890).

Hökfelt, T., Dahlström, A.: Effects of two mitosis inhibitors (colchicine and vinblastine) on the distribution and axonal transport of noradrenaline storage particles, studied by fluorescence and electron microscopy. Z. Zellforsch. **119**, 460–482 (1971).

Hoffman, H.: Acceleration and retardation of the process of axon-sprouting in partially denervated muscles. Aust. J. exp. Biol. med. Sci. **30**, 541–566 (1952).

Hoffman, H., Grigg, G. W.: An electron microscopic study of mitochondria formation. Exp. Cell Res. **15**, 118–131 (1958).

Hollande, E.: Formation et interprétation de l'appareil de Golgi: les glandes multifides de Helix pomatia L. Ann. Embryol. Morphogenèse **3**, 447–456 (1970).

Holman, J.: Occurrence and ultrastructure of lipid droplets in the developing chick intestinal epithelium. Acta anat. (Basel) **74**, 54–64 (1969).

Holtzman, E., Peterson, E. R.: Uptake of protein by mammalian neurons. J. Cell Biol. **40**, 863–869 (1969).

Hudson, G., Hartmann, J. F.: The relationship between dense bodies and mitochondria in motor neurones. Z. Zellforsch. **54**, 147–157 (1961).

Hughes, A.: The growth of embryonic neurites. A study on cultures of chick neural tissues. J. Anat. (Lond.) **87**, 150–162 (1953).

Hughes, A.: The development of the neural tube of the chick embryo. A study with the ultraviolet microscope. J. Embryol. exp. Morph. **3**, 305–325 (1955).

Huneeus, F. C., Davison, P. F.: Fibrillar proteins from squid axons. I. Neurofilament protein. J. molec. Biol. **52**, 415–428 (1970).

Hydén, H.: Protein metabolism in the nerve cell during growth and function. Acta physiol. scand. **6**, Suppl. **17**, 1–136 (1943).

James, K. A. C., Bray, J. J., Morgan, I. G., Austin, L.: The effect of colchicine on the transport of axonal protein in the chicken. Biochem. J. **117**, 767–771 (1970).

Jones, D. S.: Studies on the origin of sheath cells and sympathetic ganglia in the chick. Anat. Rec. **73**, 343–357 (1939).

Jones, E. G., Powell, T. P. S.: Synapses on the axon hillocks and initial segments of pyramidal cell axons in the cerebral cortex. J. Cell Sci. **5**, 495–507 (1969).

Karasaki, S.: Electron microscopic studies on cytoplasmic structures of ectoderm cells of the triturus embryo during the early phase of differentiation. Embryologia (Nagoya) **4**, 247–272 (1959).

Karlsson, J.-O., Sjöstrand, J.: The effect of colchicine on the axonal transport of protein in the optic nerve and tract of the rabbit. Brain Res. **13**, 617–619 (1969).

Kása, P.: Acetylcholinesterase transport in the central and peripheral nervous tissue: the role of tubules in the enzyme transport. Nature (Lond.) **218**, 1265–1267 (1968).

Kása, P., Csillik, B.: AChE synthesis in cholinergic neurons: electron histochemistry of enzyme translocation. Histochemie **12**, 175–183 (1968).

Kawana, E., Sandri, C., Akert, K.: Ultrastructure of growth cones in the cerebellar cortex of the neonatal rat and cat. Z. Zellforsch. **115**, 284–298 (1971).

Kessel, R. G.: Electron microscope studies on oocytes of an echinoderm, Thyone briareus, with special reference to the origin and structure of the annulate lamellae. J. Ultrastruct. Res. **10**, 498–514 (1964).

Kessel, R. G.: An electron microscope study of spermiogenesis in the grasshopper with particular reference to the development of microtubular systems during differentiation. J. Ultrastruct. Res. **18**, 677–694 (1967).

Kessel, R. G.: An electron microscope study of differentiation and growth in oocytes of Ophioderma panamensis. J. Ultrastruct. Res. **22**, 63–89 (1968).

Kessel, R. G.: Origin of the Golgi apparatus in embryonic cells of the grasshopper. J. Ultrastruct. Res. **34**, 260–275 (1971).

Kessel, R. G., Eichler, V. B.: Microtubules in the microspikes and cortical cytoplasm of grasshopper embryonic cells. J. Microscopie **5**, 781–786 (1966).

Kiermayer, O.: Elektronenmikroskopische Untersuchungen zum Problem der Cytomorphogenese von Micrasterias denticulata Bréb. I. Allgemeiner Überblick. Protoplasma (Wien) **69**, 97–132 (1970).

Knowles, F., Vollrath, L.: Synaptic contacts between neurosecretory fibres and pituicytes in the pituitary of the eel. Nature (Lond.) **206**, 1168–1169 (1965).

Koelle, G. B.: The histochemical identification of acetylcholinesterase in cholinergic, adrenergic and sensory neurons. J. Pharmacol. exp. Ther. **114**, 167–184 (1955).

Koelle, G. B.: Cytological distributions and physiological functions of cholinesterases. In: Handbuch der experimentellen Pharmakologie, edit. O. Eichler and A. Farah, vol. 15, p. 187–298. Berlin: Springer-Verlag 1963.

Kölliker, A.: Die Entwicklung der Elemente des Nervensystems. Z. wiss. Zool. **82**, 1–38 (1905).

Koenig, E.: Synthetic mechanisms in the axon. I. Local axonal synthesis of acetylcholinesterase. J. Neurochem. **12**, 343–355 (1965).

Koenig, E., Koelle, G. B.: Mode of regeneration of acetylcholinesterase in cholinergic neurons following irreversible inactivation. J. Neurochem. **8**, 169–188 (1961).

Kohn, A.: Über die Scheidenzellen (Randzellen) peripherer Ganglienzellen. Anat. Anz. **30**, 154–159 (1907).

Kolster, R.: Beiträge zur Kenntnis der Histogenese der peripheren Nerven nebst Bemerkungen über die Regeneration derselben nach Verletzungen. Beitr. path. Anat. **26**, 190–201 (1899).

Kornguth, S. E., Tomasi, L. G.: Changes in the distribution of a histone in dorsal root ganglion neurons during development. J. Cell Biol. **38**, 515–522 (1968).

Kreutzberg, G. W.: Neuronal dynamics and axonal flow. IV. Blockage of intra-axonal enzyme transport by colchicine. Proc. nat. Acad. Sci. (Wash.) **62**, 722–728 (1969).

Kuntz, A.: Experimental studies on the histogenesis of the sympathetic nervous system. J. comp. Neurol. **34**, 1–36 (1922).

Kwan, K.: Development of Golgi apparatus of spinal ganglion cells in rabbit. Okayima Igakkai Zasshi **48**, 2091–2092 (1936).

Lafontaine, J. G., Allard, C.: A light and electron microscope study of the morphological changes induced in rat liver cells by the azo dye 2-Me-DAB. J. Cell Biol. **22**, 143–172 (1964).

Lampert, P. W.: A comparative electron microscopic study of reactive, degenerating, regenerating, and dystrophic axons. J. Neuropath. exp. Neurol. **26**, 345–368 (1967).

Lansing, A. I., Hillier, J., Rosenthal, T. B.: Electron microscopy of some marine egg inclusions. Biol. Bull. **103**, 294 (1952).

Lanzavecchia, G., Le Coultre, A.: Origine dei mitocondri durante lo sviluppo embrionale di Rana esculenta. Studio al microscopio elettronico. Arch. ital. Anat. Embriol. **63**, 445–458 (1958).

Lanzavecchia, G., Mangioni, C.: Moltiplicazione dei mitocondri in oociti di Xenopus laevis D. Istituto Lombardo (Rend. Sci.) B **97**, 341–365 (1963).

Lasek, R.: Axoplasmic transport in cat dorsal root ganglion cells: as studied with [³H]-L-leucine. Brain Res. **7**, 360–377 (1968).

Lasher, R., Matthews, D., Whitlock, D. G.: Axoplasmic transport in cultured chick embryo sensory neurons. J. Cell Biol. **47**, 116A (1970).

LaVelle, A.: Nucleolar and Nissl substance development in nerve cells. J. comp. Neurol. **104**, 175–205 (1956).

Ledbetter, M. C., Porter, K. R.: A "microtubule" in plant cell fine structure. J. Cell Biol. **19**, 239–250 (1963).

Lehmann, F. E.: Further studies on the morphogenetic rôle of the somites in the development of the nervous system of amphibians. J. exp. Zool. **49**, 93–131 (1927).

Lenhossék, M. v.: Die Entwickelung der Ganglienanlagen bei dem menschlichen Embryo. Arch. Anat. u. Physiol., Anat. Abt., 1–25 (1891).

Lenhossék, M. v.: Beobachtungen an den Spinalganglien und dem Rückenmark von Pristiurusembryonen. Anat. Anz. **7**, 519–539 (1892).

Lenhossék, M. v.: Zur Kenntnis der Spinalganglienzellen. Arch. mikr. Anat. **69**, 245–263 (1907).

Lentz, T. L.: The fine structure of differentiating interstitial cells in Hydra. Z. Zellforsch. **67**, 547–560 (1965).

Lentz, T. L.: Fine structure of nerves in the regenerating limb of the newt Triturus. Amer. J. Anat. **121**, 647–670 (1967).

Lever, J. D.: Physiologically induced changes in adrenocortical mitochondria. J. biophys. biochem. Cytol. **2** Suppl., 313–318 (1956).

Levi, G.: La capsula delle cellule dei gangli sensitivi. Penetrazione di fibre collagene nel loro protoplasma. Monit. zool. ital. **18**, 153–158 (1907).

Levi, G.: I gangli cerebrospinali. Arch. ital. Anat. Embriol. **7** Suppl., 1–394 (1908).

Levi, G.: Connessioni e struttura degli elementi nervosi sviluppati fuori dell'organismo. Atti Reale Accad. Lincei, S. V, Cl. Sc. fis., mat. e nat. **12**, 142–182 (1917).

Lewis, M. R., Lewis, W. H.: Mitochondria (and other cytoplasmic structures) in tissue culture. Amer. J. Anat. **17**, 339–401 (1915).

Lewis, P. R., Hughes, A. F. W.: The cholinesterase of developing neurones in Xenopus laevis. In: Metabolism of the nervous system, edit. D. Richter, p. 511–514. London-New York-Paris-Los Angeles: Pergamon Press 1957.

Lewis, P. R., Shute, C. C. D.: The distribution of cholinesterase in cholinergic neurons demonstrated with the electron microscope. J. Cell Sci. **1**, 381–390 (1966).

Linnane, A. W., Vitols, E., Nowland, P. G.: Studies on the origin of yeast mitochondria. J. Cell Biol. **13**, 345–350 (1962).

Locke, M.: Cellular membranes in development. New York and London: Academic Press 1964.

Longo, F. J., Anderson, E.: Cytological events leading to the formation of the two-cell stage in the rabbit: association of the maternally and paternally derived genomes. J. Ultrastruct. Res. 29, 86–118 (1969).

Low, F. N.: Interstitial bodies in the early chick embryo. Amer. J. Anat. 128, 45–56 (1970).

Lubińska, L., Niemierko, S., Oderfeld, B., Szwarc, L.: The distribution of acetylcholinesterase in peripheral nerves. J. Neurochem. 10, 25–41 (1963).

Lubińska, L., Niemierko, S., Oderfeld-Nowak, B., Szwarc, L.: Behaviour of acetylcholinesterase in isolated nerve segments. J. Neurochem. 11, 493–503 (1964).

Luck, D. J. L.: Formation of mitochondria in Neurospora crassa. J. Cell Biol. 16, 483–499 (1963).

Luck, D. J. L.: Formation of mitochondria in Neurospora crassa. J. Cell Biol. 24, 461–470 (1965).

Lund, H. A., Vatter, A. E., Hanson, J. B.: Biochemical and cytological changes accompanying growth and differentiation in the roots of Zea mays. J. biophys. biochem. Cytol. 4, 87–98 (1958).

Lyser, K. M.: Early differentiation of motor neuroblasts in the chick embryo as studied by electron microscopy. I. General aspects. Develop. Biol. 10, 433–466 (1964).

Lyser, K. M.: Early differentiation of motor neuroblasts in the chick embryo as studied by electron microscopy. II. Microtubules and neurofilaments. Develop. Biol. 17, 117–142 (1968a).

Lyser, K. M.: An electron-microscope study of centrioles in differentiating motor neuroblasts. J. Embryol. exp. Morph. 20, 343–354 (1968b).

Lyser, K. M.: Microtubules and filaments in developing axons and optic stalk cells. Tissue and Cell 3, 395–404 (1971).

Maltzahn, K. v., Mühlethaler, K.: Observations on division of mitochondria in dedifferentiating cells of Splachnum ampullaceum (L.) Hedw. Experientia (Basel) 18, 315–316 (1962).

Manasek, F. J.: Mitosis in developing cardiac muscle. J. Cell Biol. 37, 191–196 (1968).

Manner, G.: Cell division and collagen synthesis in cultured fibroblasts. Exp. Cell Res. 65, 49–60 (1971).

Maraldi, N. M., Barbieri, M.: Ribosome crystallization. I. Study on electron microscope of ribosome crystallization during chick embryo development. J. submicr. Cytol. 1, 159–170 (1969).

Marchisio, P. C., Consolo, S.: Developmental changes of choline acetyltransferase (ChAc) activity in chick embryo spinal and sympathetic ganglia. J. Neurochem. 15, 759–764 (1968).

Marcora, F.: Über die Histogenese des Zentralnervensystems mit besonderer Rücksicht auf die innere Struktur der Nervenelemente. Folia neuro-biol. (Lpz.) 5, 928–960 (1911).

Marshall, A. M.: On the early stages of development of the nerves in birds. J. Anat. Physiol. 11, 491–515 (1877).

Marshall, A. M.: The development of the cranial nerves in the chick. Quart. J. micr. Sci. 69 (N. S. 18), 10–40 (1878).

Mayor, D., Tomlinson, D. R., Banks, P., Mraz, P.: Microtubules and the intra-axonal transport of noradrenaline storage (dense cored) vesicles. J. Anat. (Lond.) 111, 344–345 (1972).

Meller, K., Breipohl, W., Glees, P.: The cytology of the developing molecular layer of mouse motor cortex. Z. Zellforsch. 86, 171–183 (1968).

Meller, K., Eschner, J., Glees, P.: The differentiation of endoplasmic reticulum in developing neurons of the chick spinal cord. Z. Zellforsch. 69, 189–197 (1966).

Meyer, H. H.: Über die Wirkung des Kalkes. Münch. med. Wschr. 57, 2277–2278 (1910).

Miller, F.: Orthologie und Pathologie der Zelle im elektronenmikroskopischen Bild. Verh. dtsch. Ges. Path. 42, 261–332 (1958).

Miller, R., Varon, S., Kruger, L., Coates, P. W., Orkand, P. M.: Formation of synaptic contacts on dissociated chick embryo sensory ganglion cells in vitro. Brain Res. 24, 356–358 (1970).

Mollenhauer, H. H., Morré, D. J.: Golgi apparatus and plant secretion. Ann. Rev. Plant Physiol. 17, 27–46 (1966).

Moore, R. T., McAlear, J. H.: Fine structure of mycota. IV. The occurrence of the Golgi dictyosome in the fungus Neobulgaria pura (Fr.) Petrak. J. Cell Biol. 16, 131–141 (1963).

Morpurgo, B., Tirelli, V.: Sur le développement des ganglions intervertébraux du lapin. Arch. ital. Biol. 18, 413–435 (1893).

Morré, J., Mollenhauer, H. H., Bracker, C. E.: Origin and continuity of Golgi apparatus. In: Origin and continuity of cell organelles, edit. J. Reinert and H. Ursprung, p. 82–126. Berlin-Heidelberg-New York: Springer 1971.

Morris, J. H., Hudson, A. R., Weddell, G.: A study of degeneration and regeneration in the divided rat sciatic nerve based on electron microscopy. IV. Changes in fascicular microtopography, perineurium and endoneurial fibroblasts. Z. Zellforsch. 124, 165–203 (1972).

Moses, M. J.: Studies on nuclei using correlated cytochemical, light, and electron microscope techniques. J. biophys. biochem. Cytol. 2 Suppl., 397–406 (1956).

Müller, E., Ingvar, S.: Über den Ursprung des Sympathicus beim Hühnchen. Arch. mikr. Anat. 99, 650–671 (1923).

Muir, A. R.: The effects of divalent cations on the ultrastructure of the perfused rat heart. J. Anat. (Lond.) 101, 239–261 (1967).

Mukerjee, H., Sri Ram, J., Pierce, G. B., Jr.: Basement membranes. V. Chemical composition of neoplastic basement membrane mucoprotein. Amer. J. Path. 46, 49–58 (1965).

Munger, B. L.: A phase and electron microscopic study of cellular differentiation in pancreatic acinar cells of the mouse. Amer. J. Anat. 103, 1–33 (1958).

Nachmansohn, D.: Chemical and molecular basis of nerve activity. New York: Academic Press 1959.

Nachmansohn, D.: Chemical factors controlling nerve activity. Science 134, 1962–1968 (1961).

Nagai, R., Rebhun, L. I.: Cytoplasmic microfilaments in streaming Nitella cells. J. Ultrastruct. Res. 14, 571–589 (1966).

Nakai, J., Kawasaki, Y.: Studies on the mechanism determining the course of nerve fibers in tissue culture. I. The reaction of the growth cone to various obstructions. Z. Zellforsch. 51, 108–122 (1959).

Nathaniel, E. J. H., Pease, D. C.: Collagen and basement membrane formation by Schwann cells during nerve regeneration. J. Ultrastruct. Res. 9, 550–560 (1963).

Newcomer, E. H.: Mitochondria in plants. Bot. Rev. 6, 85–147 (1940).

Niklowitz, W., Bak, I. J.: Elektronenmikroskopische Untersuchungen am Ammonshorn. I. Die normale Substruktur der Pyramidenzellen. Z. Zellforsch. 66, 529–547 (1965).

Norberg, H. S.: The follicular oocyte and its granulosa cells in domestic pig. Z. Zellforsch. 131, 497–517 (1972).

Oberling, C.: The structure of cytoplasm. Int. Rev. Cytol. 8, 1–31 (1959).

Oberpriller, J. O., Oberpriller, J. C.: Mitosis in adult newt ventricle. J. Cell Biol. 49, 560–563 (1971).

Ochoa, J., Vial, J. D.: Behaviour of peripheral nerve structures in chronic neuropathies, with special reference to the Schwann cell. J. Anat. (Lond.) 102, 95–111 (1967).

Olivo, O. M., Porta, E., Barberis, L.: Ricerche sulla velocità di accrescimento delle cellule e degli organi. IV. Modalità di accrescimento delle cellule dei gangli spinali nel pollo durante la vita embrionale e postnatale. Arch. ital. Anat. Embriol. 30, 34–71 (1932).

Onodi, A. D.: Über die Entwickelung der Spinalganglien und der Nervenwurzeln. Int. Mschr. Anat. Physiol. 1, 204–209, 255–284 (1884).

Orr, D. W., Windle, W. F.: The development of behavior in chick embryos: the appearance of somatic movements. J. comp. Neurol. 60, 271–285 (1934).

Orrenius, S., Ericsson, J. L. E.: Enzyme-membrane relationship in phenobarbital induction of synthesis of drug-metabolizing enzyme system and proliferation of endoplasmic membranes. J. Cell Biol. 28, 181–198 (1966).

Overton, J.: Desmosome development in normal and reassociating cells in the early chick blastoderm. Develop. Biol. 4, 532–548 (1962).

Ovtracht, L.: Morphogenèse des dictyosomes dans des cellules sécrétrices à cycle sécrétoire saisonnier. J. Microscopie 11, 84–85 (1971).

Palay, S. L., Palade, G. E.: The fine structure of neurons. J. biophys. biochem. Cytol. 1, 69–88 (1955).

Palay, S. L., Sotelo, C., Peters, A., Orkand, P. M.: The axon hillock and the initial segment. J. Cell Biol. 38, 193–201 (1968).

Palladini, G.: Neurodegenerazione nella ontogenesi di quaglia (Coturnix coturnix japonica T. e S.). Riv. Neurobiol. (Arezzo) 7, 383–400 (1961).

Pannese, E.: Observations on the ultrastructure of the enamel organ. III. Internal and external enamel epithelia. J. Ultrastruct. Res. 6, 186–204 (1962).

Pannese, E.: Structures possibly related to the formation of new mitochondria in spinal ganglion neuroblasts. J. Ultrastruct. Res. 15, 57–65 (1966a).

Pannese, E.: Expansive growth of the nuclear envelope and formation of mitochondria in ganglionic neuroblasts. Z. Zellforsch. 72, 295–324 (1966b).

Pannese, E.: Membranous structures in continuity with the nuclear envelope, in neuroblasts. Acta Embryol. Morph. exp. (Palermo) 9, 69–76 (1966c).

Pannese, E.: Developmental changes of the endoplasmic reticulum and ribosomes in nerve cells of the spinal ganglia of the domestic fowl. J. comp. Neurol. 132, 331–364 (1968a).

Pannese, E.: Temporary junctions between neuroblasts in the developing spinal ganglia of the domestic fowl. J. Ultrastruct. Res. 21, 233–250 (1968b).

Pannese, E.: Electron microscopical study on the development of the satellite cell sheath in spinal ganglia. J. comp. Neurol. 135, 381–422 (1969).

Pannese, E., Bianchi, R., Calligaris, B., Ventura, R., Weibel, E. R.: Quantitative relationships between nerve and satellite cells in spinal ganglia. An electron microscopical study. I. Mammals. Brain Res. 46, 215–234 (1972).

Pannese, E., Luciano, L., Iurato, S., Reale, E.: Histochemical localization of acetylcholinesterase (AChE) activity in embryonic spinal ganglion neuroblasts. 7th Int. Congr. Electr. Micr. Grenoble 3, 695–696 (1970).

Pannese, E., Luciano, L., Iurato, S., Reale, E.: Cholinesterase activity in spinal ganglia neuroblasts: a histochemical study at the electron microscope. J. Ultrastruct. Res. 36, 46–67 (1971).

Pannese, E., Luciano, L., Iurato, S., Reale, E.: The localization of acetylcholinesterase activity in the spinal ganglia of the adult fowl studied by electron microscope histochemistry. Histochemistry, in press (1974).

Parks, H. F.: Unusual formations of ergastoplasm in parotid acinous cells of mice. J. Cell Biol. 14, 221–234 (1962).

Pasteels, J. J., Castiaux, P., Vandermeerssche, G.: Ultrastructure du cytoplasme et distribution de l'acide ribonucleique dans l'oeuf fecondé, tant normal que centrifugé de Paracentrotus lividus. Arch. Biol. (Liège) 69, 627–643 (1959).

Peachey, L. D.: Electron microscopic observations on the accumulation of divalent cations in intramitochondrial granules. J. Cell Biol. 20, 95–111 (1964).

Peters, A.: A stellate cell axon in the rat cerebral cortex. Anat. Rec. 169, 400 (1971).

Peters, A., Muir, A. R.: The relationship between axons and Schwann cells during development of peripheral nerves in the rat. Quart. J. exp. Physiol. 46, 117–130 (1959).

Peters, A., Proskauer, C. C., Kaiserman-Abramof, I. R: The small pyramidal neuron of the rat cerebral cortex. The axon hillock and initial segment. J. Cell Biol. 39, 604–619 (1968).

Peters, A., Vaughn, J. E.: Microtubules and filaments in the axons and astrocytes of early postnatal rat optic nerves. J. Cell Biol. 32, 113–119 (1967).

Peterson, E. R., Murray, M. R.: Myelin sheath formation in cultures of avian spinal ganglia. Amer. J. Anat. 96, 319–355 (1955).

Peterson, E. R., Murray, M. R.: Modification of development in isolated dorsal root ganglia by nutritional and physical factors. Develop. Biol. 2, 461–476 (1960).

Pierce, G. B., Jr.: The epithelial origin of basement membranes. J. Cell Biol. 23, 74A (1964).

Pierce, G. B., Jr.: The development of basement membranes of the mouse embryo. Develop. Biol. 13, 231–249 (1966).

Pierce, G. B., Jr., Beals, T. F., Sri Ram, J., Midgley, A. R.: Basement membranes. IV. Epithelial origin and immunologic cross reactions. Amer. J. Path. 45, 929–961 (1964).

Pierce, G. B., Jr., Midgley, A. R., Jr., Sri Ram, J., Feldman, J. D.: Parietal yolk sac carcinoma: clue to the histogenesis of Reichert's membrane of the mouse embryo. Amer. J. Path. 41, 549–566 (1962).

Pilati, L.: Statistische Untersuchungen über das Wachstum der Nervenzellen der menschlichen Spinalganglien. Z. mikr.-anat. Forsch. 44, 1–32 (1938).

Pollard, T. D., Ito, S.: Cytoplasmic filaments of Amoeba proteus. I. The role of filaments in consistency changes and movement. J. Cell Biol. 46, 267–289 (1970).

Pomerat, C. M., Hendelman, W. J., Raiborn, C. W., Jr., Massey, J. F.: Dynamic activities of nervous tissue in vitro. In: The neuron, edit. H. Hydén, p. 119–178. Amsterdam-London-New York: Elsevier Publ. Co. 1967.

Porter, K. R.: The ground substance; observations from electron microscopy. In: The cell, edit. J. Brachet and A. E. Mirsky, vol. 2, p. 621–675. New York and London: Academic Press 1961.

Porter, K. R.: Cytoplasmic microtubules and their functions. In: Principles of biomolecular organization, p. 308–356. The Ciba Foundation Symp. London: J. & A. Churchill Ltd. 1966.

Potter, D. D., Furshpan, E. J., Lennox, E. S.: Connections between cells of the developing squid as revealed by electrophysiological methods. Proc. nat. Acad. Sci. (Wash.) 55, 328–335 (1966).

Prestige, M. C.: Cell turnover in the spinal ganglia of Xenopus laevis tadpoles. J. Embryol. exp. Morph. 13, 63–72 (1965).

Preyer, W.: Spezielle Physiologie des Embryo. Leipzig: Grieben 1885.

Priest, R. E., Davies, L. M.: Cellular proliferation and synthesis of collagen. Lab. Invest. 21, 138–142 (1969).

Przybylski, R. J.: Occurrence of centrioles during skeletal and cardiac myogenesis. J. Cell Biol. 48, 214–221 (1971).

Radouco-Thomas, C., Nosal, Gl., Radouco-Thomas, S.: The nuclear-ribosomal system during neuronal differentiation and development. In: Chemistry and brain development, edit. R. Paoletti and A. N. Davison, p. 291–308. New York: Plenum Press 1971.

Rau, A. S., Ludford, R. J.: Variations in the form of the Golgi bodies during the development of neurones. Quart. J. micr. Sci. 69, 509–518 (1925).

Raven, Chr. P.: Experiments on the origin of the sheath cells and sympathetic neuroblasts in Amphibia. J. comp. Neurol. 67, 221–240 (1937).

Remak, R.: Untersuchungen über die Entwickelung der Wirbelthiere. Berlin 1851.

Retzius, G.: Zur Kenntniss der Ependymzellen der Centralorgane. Verh. biol. Ver. (Stockh.) 3, 103–116 (1891).

Revel, J. P., Karnovsky, M. J.: Hexagonal array of subunits in intercellular junctions of the mouse heart and liver. J. Cell Biol. 33, C7–C12 (1967).

Rhea, R. P.: Electron microscopic observations on the slime mold Physarum polycephalum with specific reference to fibrillar structures. J. Ultrastruct. Res. 15, 349–379 (1966).

Robertson, J. D.: The function and metabolism of calcium in the Invertebrates. Biol. Rev. 16, 106 (1941).

Robertson, J. D.: The ultrastructure of cell membranes and their derivatives. Biochem. Soc. Symp. 16, 3–43 (1959).

Rosenbluth, J.: Subsurface cisterns and their relationship to the neuronal plasma membrane. J. Cell Biol. 13, 405–422 (1962).

Rosenbluth, J., Wissig, S. L.: The distribution of exogenous ferritin in toad spinal ganglia and the mechanism of its uptake by neurons. J. Cell Biol. 23, 307–325 (1964).

Roth, L. E.: An electron microscope study of the cytology of the protozoan Euplotes patella. J. biophys. biochem. Cytol. 3, 985–1000 (1957).

Roth, T. F., Porter, K. R.: Yolk protein uptake in the oocyte of the mosquito Aedes aegypti L. J. Cell Biol. 20, 313–332 (1964).

Rouiller, C., Bernhard, W.: "Microbodies" and the problem of mitochondrial regeneration in liver cells. J. biophys. biochem. Cytol. 2 Suppl., 355–360 (1956).

Rouiller, C., Simon, G.: Contribution de la microscopie électronique au progrès de nos connaissances en cytologie et en histo-pathologie hépatique. Rev. int. Hépat. 12, 167–206 (1962).

Ruby, J. R., Webster, R. M.: Origin of the Golgi complex in germ cells in the developing ovary of the bat. Z. Zellforsch. 133, 1–12 (1972).

Rumyantsev, P. P., Snigirevskaya, E. S.: The ultrastructure of differentiating cells of the heart muscle in the state of mitotic division. Acta morph. Acad. Sci. hung. 16, 271–283 (1968).

Sabnis, D. D., Jacobs, W. P.: Cytoplasmic streaming and microtubules in the coenocytic marine alga, Caulerpa prolifera. J. Cell Sci. 2, 465–472 (1967).

Saunders, J. W., Jr.: Death in embryonic systems. Science 154, 604–612 (1966).

Sawyer, C. H.: Cholinesterase and the behavior problem in Amblystoma. I. The relationship between the development of the enzyme and early motility. II. The effects of inhibiting cholinesterase. J. exp. Zool. 92, 1–29 (1943).

Saxod, R.: Etude au microscope électronique de l'histogenèse du corpuscule sensoriel cutané de Herbst chez le Canard. J. Ultrastruct. Res. **33**, 463–482 (1970).

Scharf, J. H.: Sensible Ganglien. In: Nervensystem. Handbuch der mikroskopischen Anatomie des Menschen, von M. v. Möllendorff u. W. Bargmann, Bd. 4/3, S. 181–188. Berlin-Göttingen-Heidelberg: Springer 1958.

Scharff, M. D., Robbins, E.: Polyribosome disaggregation during metaphase. Science **151**, 992–995 (1966).

Scharrer, B., Wurzelmann, S.: Ultrastructural study on nuclear-cytoplasmic relationships in oocytes of the African lungfish, Protopterus aethiopicus. I. Nucleolo-cytoplasmic pathways. Z. Zellforsch. **96**, 325–343 (1969a).

Scharrer, B., Wurzelmann, S.: Ultrastructural study on nuclear-cytoplasmic relationships in oocytes of the African lungfish, Protopterus aethiopicus. II. The microtubular apparatus of the nuclear envelope. Z. Zellforsch. **101**, 1–12 (1969b).

Schjeide, O. A., McCandless, R. G.: On the formation of mitochondria. Growth **26**, 309–321 (1962).

Schjeide, O. A., McCandless, R. G., Munn, R. J.: Mitochondrial morphogenesis. Nature (Lond.) **203**, 158–160 (1964).

Schlaepfer, W. W.: Acetylcholinesterase activity of motor and sensory nerve fibers in the spinal nerve roots of the rat. Z. Zellforsch. **88**, 441–456 (1968).

Schmitt, F. O.: Fibrous proteins—neuronal organelles. Proc. nat. Acad. Sci. (Wash.) **60**, 1092–1101 (1968).

Schmitt, F. O.: Fibrous proteins and neuronal dynamics. In: Cellular dynamics of the neuron, edit. S. H. Barondes, p. 95–111. New York and London: Academic Press 1969.

Schmitt, F. O., Samson, F. E., Jr.: Neuronal fibrous proteins. Neurosci. Res. Prog. Bull. **6**, 113–219 (1968).

Schochet, S. S., Jr.: Mitochondrial changes in axonal dystrophy produced by vitamin E deficiency. Acta neuropath. (Berl.) Suppl. 5, 54–60 (1971).

Sechrist, J. W.: Neurocytogenesis. I. Neurofibrils, neurofilaments, and the terminal mitotic cycle. Amer. J. Anat. **124**, 117–134 (1969).

Sedar, A. W., Forte, J. G.: Effects of calcium depletion on the junctional complex between oxyntic cells of gastric glands. J. Cell Biol. **22**, 173–188 (1964).

Selwood, L.: Electron microscopy of the fate of exogenous ferritin in the feline visual cortex. Z. Zellforsch. **107**, 6–14 (1970).

Sjöstrand, J.: Axoplasmic transport in peripheral nerves. Exp. Cell Res. **58**, 461 (1969).

Slautterback, D. B.: Cytoplasmic microtubules. I. Hydra. J. Cell Biol. **18**, 367–388 (1963).

Slautterback, D. B., Fawcett, D. W.: The development of the cnidoblasts of Hydra. An electron microscope study of cell differentiation. J. biophys. biochem. Cytol. **5**, 441–452 (1959).

Sobkowicz, H. M., Hartmann, H. A., Monzain, R., Desnoyers, P.: Growth, differentiation and ribonucleic acid content of the fetal rat spinal ganglion cells in culture. J. comp. Neurol. **148**, 249–284 (1973).

Spassova, I.: Ultrastructure of the encapsulated nerve endings in the lips of the cat. J. submicr. Cytol. **3**, 339–352 (1971).

Speidel, C. C.: Studies of living nerves. II. Activities of ameboid growth cones, sheath cells, and myelin segments, as revealed by prolonged observation of individual nerve fibers in frog tadpoles. Amer. J. Anat. **52**, 1–79 (1933).

Stang-Voss, C.: Zur Entstehung des Golgi-Apparates. Elektronenmikroskopische Untersuchungen an Spermatiden von Eisenia foetida (Annelidae). Z. Zellforsch. **109**, 287–296 (1970).

Stang-Voss, C., Staubesand, J.: Über die Neubildung von Mitochondrien. Elektronenmikroskopische Untersuchungen an Spermatiden von Eisenia foetida (Annelidae). Z. Zellforsch. **111**, 127–142 (1970).

Stäubli, W., Freyvogel, T. A., Suter, J.: Structural modification of the endoplasmic reticulum of midgut epithelial cells of mosquitoes in relation to blood intake. J. Microscopie **5**, 189–204 (1966).

Stefanelli, A.: Nuovi aspetti e considerazioni sulla citomorfosi delle cellule nervose. Ric. Sci. **25**, 2778–2795 (1955).

Streeter, G. L.: On the histogenesis of spinal ganglia in mammals. Amer. J. Anat. 4, XIII (1905).

Streeter, G. L.: The development of the nervous system. In: Manual of human embryology, edit. F. Keibel and F. P. Mall, vol. 2, p. 1–156. Philadelphia and London: J. B. Lippincott Co. 1912.

Stroganova, N. S., Monakhova, M. A.: The formation of mitochondria from the cell wall in spermatogonia of the grain mite. Dokl. Akad. Nauk SSSR 160, 937–939 (1965).

Strumia, E., Baima-Bollone, P. L.: AChE activity in the spinal ganglia of the chick embryo during development. Acta anat. (Basel) 57, 281–293 (1964).

Taddei, C.: Ribosome arrangement during oogenesis of Lacerta sicula Raf. Exp. Cell Res. 70, 285–292 (1972).

Tahmisian, T. N., Powers, E. L., Devine, R. L.: Light and electron microscope studies of morphological changes of mitochondria during spermatogenesis in the grasshopper. J. biophys. biochem. Cytol. 2 Suppl., 325–330 (1956).

Tandler, B., Erlandson, R. A., Smith, A. L., Wynder, E. L.: Riboflavin and mouse hepatic cell structure and function. II. Division of mitochondria during recovery from simple deficiency. J. Cell Biol. 41, 477–493 (1969).

Tandler, B., Moriber, L. G.: Microtubular structures associated with the acrosome during spermiogenesis in the water-strider, Gerris remigis (Say). J. Ultrastruct. Res. 14, 391–404 (1966).

Taxi, J.: Contribution a l'étude des connexions des neurones moteurs du système nerveux autonome. Ann. Sci. nat. Zool. 7, 413–674 (1965).

Taylor, E. W.: Contractile proteins and cytoplasmic movement. Neurosci. Res. Prog. Bull. 5, 333–337 (1967).

Tello, F.: Las neurofibrillas en los vertebrados inferiores. Trav. Lab. Invest. Biol. Univ. Madrid 3, 113–151 (1904).

Tennyson, V. M.: Electron microscopic study of the developing neuroblast of the dorsal root ganglion of the rabbit embryo. J. comp. Neurol. 124, 267–318 (1965).

Tennyson, V. M.: The fine structure of the axon and growth cone of the dorsal root neuroblast of the rabbit embryo. J. Cell Biol. 44, 62–79 (1970a).

Tennyson, V. M.: The fine structure of the developing nervous system. In: Developmental neurobiology, edit. W. A. Himwich, p. 47–116. Springfield, Ill.: Ch. C. Thomas 1970b.

Tennyson, V. M., Brzin, M.: Electron microscopic and micro-gasometric studies of cholinesterase development in embryonic dorsal root neuroblasts. Anat. Rec. 160, 440 (1968).

Tennyson, V. M., Brzin, M.: The appearance of acetylcholinesterase in the dorsal root neuroblast of the rabbit embryo. A study by electron microscope cytochemistry and microgasometric analysis with the magnetic diver. J. Cell Biol. 46, 64–80 (1970).

Tennyson, V. M., Brzin, M., Duffy, P. E.: Cholinesterase localization in the dorsal root ganglion of the rabbit embryo by electron microscopic histochemistry. J. Neuropath. exp. Neurol. 26, 136 (1967).

Thomas, P. K.: The deposition of collagen in relation to Schwann cell basement membrane during peripheral nerve regeneration. J. Cell Biol. 23, 375–382 (1964).

Threadgold, L. T., Lasker, R.: Mitochondriogenesis in integumentary cells of the larval sardine (Sardinops caerulea). J. Ultrastruct. Res. 19, 238–249 (1967).

Tilney, L. G., Gibbins, J. R.: Microtubules and filaments in the filopodia of the secondary mesenchyme cells of Arbacia punctulata and Echinarachnius parma. J. Cell Sci. 5, 195–210 (1969).

Tilney, L. G., Hiramoto, Y., Marsland, D.: Studies on the microtubules in Heliozoa. III. A pressure analysis of the role of these structures in the formation and maintenance of the axopodia of Actinosphaerium nucleofilum (Barrett). J. Cell Biol. 29, 77–95 (1966).

Tilney, L. G., Porter, K. R.: Studies on microtubules in Heliozoa. I. The fine structure of Actinosphaerium nucleofilum (Barrett), with particular reference to the axial rod structure. Protoplasma (Wien) 60, 317–344 (1965).

Tilney, L. G., Porter, K. R.: Studies on microtubules in Heliozoa. II. The effect of low temperature on these structures in the formation and maintenance of the axopodia. J. Cell Biol. 34, 327–343 (1967).

Timofeew, D.: Beobachtungen über den Bau der Nervenzellen der Spinalganglien und des Sympathicus beim Vogel. Int. Mschr. Anat. Physiol. 15, 259–268 (1898).

Turbes, C. C.: Neuroplasmic flow studies on the peripheral and central process of the dorsal root ganglion cells. Anat. Rec. 166, 391 (1970).

Villegas, G. M., Villegas, R.: Extracellular pathways in the peripheral nerve fibres: Schwann-cell-layer permeability to thorium dioxide. Biochim. biophys. Acta (Amst.) 88, 231–233 (1964).

Visintini, F., Levi-Montalcini, R.: Relazione tra differenziazione strutturale e funzionale dei centri e delle vie nervose nell'embrione di pollo. Schweiz. Arch. Neurol. Psychiat. 43/44, 1–45 (1939).

Vivier, E., Schrevel, J.: Les ultrastructures cytoplasmiques de Selenidium hollandei, n. sp. Grégarine parasite de Sabellaria alveolata L. J. Microscopie 5, 213–228 (1966).

Wallace, P. G., Linnane, A. W.: Oxygen-induced synthesis of yeast mitochondria. Nature (Lond.) 201, 1191–1194 (1964).

Ward, R. T., Ward, E.: The multiplication of Golgi bodies in the oocytes of Rana pipiens. J. Microscopie 7, 1007–1020 (1968).

Wechsler, W.: Elektronenmikroskopische Untersuchungen der Entwicklung von Nervenzellen und Nervenfasern bei Hühnerembryonen. Anat. Anz. Erg.-H. zu 115, 287–302 (1965).

Wechsler, W., Hager, H.: Elektronenmikroskopische Befunde zur Feinstruktur von Axon-veränderungen im proximalen Stumpf regenerierenden Nn. ischiadici der weissen Ratte. Deutsche Gesellschaft für Elektronenmikroskopie (10. Tagg. 1961, Kiel) Programm und Autorenreferate, p. 38–40.

Weinstein, R. B., Hay, E. D.: Deoxyribonucleic acid synthesis and mitosis in differentiated cardiac muscle cells of chick embryos. J. Cell Biol. 47, 310–316 (1970).

Weis, P.: Confronting subsurface cisternae in chick embryo spinal ganglia. J. Cell Biol. 39, 485–488 (1968).

Weis, P.: The in vitro effect of the nerve growth factor on chick embryo spinal ganglia: an electron microscopic evaluation. J. comp. Neurol. 141, 117–132 (1971).

Weissenfels, N.: Über die Entleerung und Entwicklung der Mitochondrien und den Feinbau des Cytoplasmas von embryonalen Zellen. Z. Naturforsch. 13b, 182–186 (1958).

Wenzel, M., Grosse, G., Tapp, R. ,Wenzel, J.: Elektronenmikroskopische Untersuchungen zur Entwicklung der Neurone in Explantatkulturen des Ganglion trigeminale beim Hühner-embryo. Z. mikr.-anat. Forsch. 87, 379–409 (1973).

Weston, J. A.: A radioautographic analysis of the migration and localization of trunk neural crest cells in the chick. Develop. Biol. 6, 279–310 (1963).

Weston, J. A.: The migration and differentiation of neural crest cells. In: Advances in morphogenesis, edit. M. Abercrombie, J. Brachet and T. J. King, vol. 8, p. 41–114. New York and London: Academic Press 1970.

Weston, J. C., Ackerman, G. A., Greider, M. H., Nikolewski, R. F.: Nuclear membrane contributions to the Golgi complex. Z. Zellforsch. 123, 153–160 (1972).

Westrum, L. E.: Observations on initial segments of axons in the prepyriform cortex of the rat. J. comp. Neurol. 139, 337–356 (1970).

Wettstein, R., Sotelo, J. R.: Electronmicroscope study on the regenerative process of peripheral nerves of mice. Z. Zellforsch. 59, 708–730 (1963).

Whaley, W. G.: Proposals concerning replication of the Golgi apparatus. In: Probleme der biologischen Reduplikation, edit. P. Sitte, p. 340–371. Berlin-Heidelberg-New York: Springer 1966.

Whaley, W. G., Kephart, J. E., Mollenhauer, H. H.: The dynamics of cytoplasmic membranes during development. In: Cellular membranes in development, edit. M. Locke, p. 135–173. New York and London: Academic Press 1964.

Windle, W. F., Orr, D. W.: The development of behavior in chick embryos: spinal cord structure correlated with early somatic motility. J. comp. Neurol. 60, 287–307 (1934).

Wischnitzer, S.: An electron microscopic study of the Golgi apparatus of amphibian oocytes. Z. Zellforsch. 57, 202–212 (1962).

Wise, G. E.: Connections between cisternae of the Golgi apparatus and the granular endoplasmic reticulum in Amoeba proteus. Z. Zellforsch. 126, 431–436 (1972).

Wisniewski, H., Shelanski, M. L., Terry, R. D.: Effects of mitotic spindle inhibitors on neuro-tubules and neurofilaments in anterior horn cells. J. Cell Biol. **38**, 224–229 (1968).

Wittkowski, W.: Zur Ultrastruktur der ependymalen Tanyzyten und Pituizyten sowie ihre synaptische Verknüpfung in der Neurohypophyse des Meerschweinchens. Acta anat. (Basel) **67**, 338–360 (1967).

Wohlfarth-Bottermann, K. E.: Cytologische Studien. IV. Die Entstehung, Vermehrung und Sekretabgabe der Mitochondrien von Paramecium. Z. Naturforsch. **12b**, 164-167 (1957).

Wohlfarth-Bottermann, K. E.: Differentiations of the ground-plasm and their significance for the generation of motile force of amoeboid movement. In: Primitive motile systems in cell biology, edit. R. D. Allen and N. Kamiya, p. 79–109. New York: Academic Press Inc. 1964.

Wohlfarth-Bottermann, K. E., Moericke, V.: Gesetzmässiges Vorkommen cytoplasmatischer Lamellensysteme in Abhängigkeit vom Funktionsrhythmus einer Zelle. Z. Naturforsch. **14b**, 446–450 (1959).

Wohlman, A., Allen, R. D.: Structural organization associated with pseudopod extension and contraction during cell locomotion in Difflugia. J. Cell Sci. **3**, 105–114 (1968).

Wuerker, R. B., Palay, S. L.: Neurofilaments and microtubules in anterior horn cells of the rat. Tissue and Cell **1**, 387–402 (1969).

Yamada, K. M., Spooner, B. S., Wessells, N. K.: Axon growth: roles of microfilaments and microtubules. Proc. nat. Acad. Sci. (Wash.) **66**, 1206–1212 (1970).

Yamada, K. M., Spooner, B. S., Wessells, N. K.: Ultrastructure and function of growth cones and axons of cultured nerve cells. J. Cell Biol. **49**, 614–635 (1971).

Yamada, K. M., Wessells, N. K.: Axon elongation. Effect of nerve growth factor on micro-tubule protein. Exp. Cell Res. **66**, 346–352 (1971).

Yamadori, T.: A light and electron microscopic study on the postnatal development of spinal ganglia in rats. Acta anat. Nippon. **45**, 191–205 (1970).

Yamamoto, K., Onozato, H.: Electron microscope study on the growing oocyte of the goldfish during the first growth phase. Mem. Fac. Fisheries, Hokkaido Univ. **13**, 79–106 (1965).

Yamamoto, T.: On the thickness of the unit membrane. J. Cell Biol. **17**, 413–421 (1963).

Yates, R. D.: A study of cell division in chick embryonic ganglia. J. exp. Zool. **147**, 167–181 (1961).

Zeigel, R. F., Dalton, A. J.: Speculations based on the morphology of the Golgi systems in several types of protein-secreting cells. J. Cell Biol. **15**, 45–54 (1962).

Zelená, J.: Ribosome-like particles in myelinated axons of the rat. Brain Res. **24**, 359–363 (1970).

Zelená, J.: Ribosomes in myelinated axons of dorsal root ganglia. Z. Zellforsch. **124**, 217–229 (1972).

Zimmermann, P.: Struktur, Verteilung und Funktion der Kontaktzonen im Bauchmark von Lumbricus terrestris L. Z. Zellforsch. **87**, 137–158 (1968).

Zollinger, H. U.: Les mitochondries. Rev. Hémat. **5**, 696–745 (1956).

Subject Index